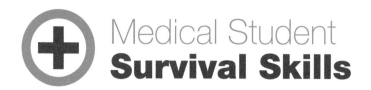

Medical Student
Survival Skills

The Acutely Ill Patient

T0131189

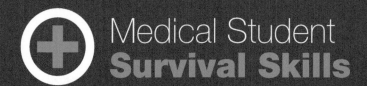

Medical Student
Survival Skills

The Acutely Ill Patient

Philip Jevon RN BSc(Hons) PGCE
Academy Manager/Tutor
Walsall Teaching Academy, Manor Hospital, Walsall, UK

Konnur Ramkumar FRCA
Consultant Anaesthetist, Senior Academy Tutor
Walsall Healthcare NHS Trust, Manor Hospital, Walsall, UK

Emma Jenkinson BSc MBChB FRCEM
Consultant, Emergency Medicine and Paediatric Emergency Medicine
The Royal Wolverhampton NHS Trust, New Cross Hospital, West Midlands, UK

Consulting Editors

Jonathan Pepper BMedSci BM BS FRCOG MD FAcadMEd
Consultant Obstetrics and Gynaecology, Head of Academy
Walsall Healthcare NHS Trust, Manor Hospital, Walsall, UK

Jamie Coleman MBChB MD MA(Med Ed) FRCP FBPhS
Professor in Clinical Pharmacology and Medical Education / MBChB Deputy
  Programme Director
School of Medicine, University of Birmingham, Birmingham, UK

WILEY Blackwell

This edition first published 2020
© 2020 by John Wiley & Sons Ltd

The right of Philip Jevon, Konnur Ramkumar, and Emma Jenkinson to be identified as the authors in this work has been asserted in accordance with law.

Registered Office(s)
John Wiley & Sons, Inc., 111 River Street, Hoboken, NJ 07030, USA
John Wiley & Sons Ltd, The Atrium, Southern Gate, Chichester, West Sussex, PO19 8SQ, UK

Editorial Office
9600 Garsington Road, Oxford, OX4 2DQ, UK

For details of our global editorial offices, customer services, and more information about Wiley products visit us at www.wiley.com.

Wiley also publishes its books in a variety of electronic formats and by print-on-demand. Some content that appears in standard print versions of this book may not be available in other formats.

Limit of Liability/Disclaimer of Warranty
The contents of this work are intended to further general scientific research, understanding, and discussion only and are not intended and should not be relied upon as recommending or promoting scientific method, diagnosis, or treatment by physicians for any particular patient. In view of ongoing research, equipment modifications, changes in governmental regulations, and the constant flow of information relating to the use of medicines, equipment, and devices, the reader is urged to review and evaluate the information provided in the package insert or instructions for each medicine, equipment, or device for, among other things, any changes in the instructions or indication of usage and for added warnings and precautions. While the publisher and authors have used their best efforts in preparing this work, they make no representations or warranties with respect to the accuracy or completeness of the contents of this work and specifically disclaim all warranties, including without limitation any implied warranties of merchantability or fitness for a particular purpose. No warranty may be created or extended by sales representatives, written sales materials or promotional statements for this work. The fact that an organization, website, or product is referred to in this work as a citation and/or potential source of further information does not mean that the publisher and authors endorse the information or services the organization, website, or product may provide or recommendations it may make. This work is sold with the understanding that the publisher is not engaged in rendering professional services. The advice and strategies contained herein may not be suitable for your situation. You should consult with a specialist where appropriate. Further, readers should be aware that websites listed in this work may have changed or disappeared between when this work was written and when it is read. Neither the publisher nor authors shall be liable for any loss of profit or any other commercial damages, including but not limited to special, incidental, consequential, or other damages.

Library of Congress Cataloging-in-Publication Data
Names: Jevon, Philip, author. | Ramkumar, Konnur, author. | Jenkinson, Emma, author.
Title: Medical student survival skills. The acutely ill patient / Philip Jevon, Konnur Ramkumar,
    Emma Jenkinson.
Other titles: Acutely ill patient
Description: Hoboken, NJ : Wiley-Blackwell, 2020. | Includes bibliographical references and index. |
Identifiers: LCCN 2018060343 (print) | LCCN 2018061628 (ebook) | ISBN 9781118902813 (Adobe PDF) |
    ISBN 9781118902820 (ePub) | ISBN 9781118902837 (pbk.)
Subjects: | MESH: Acute Disease | Emergencies | Handbook
Classification: LCC RC86.7 (ebook) | LCC RC86.7 (print) | NLM WB 39 | DDC 616.02/5–dc23
LC record available at https://lccn.loc.gov/2018060343

Cover Design: Wiley
Cover Image: © LolitaDesign/Shutterstock

Set in 9.25/12.5pt Helvetica Neue by SPi Global, Pondicherry, India

Printed in Great Britain by TJ International Ltd, Padstow, Cornwall

10 9 8 7 6 5 4 3 2 1

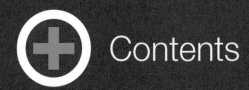

Contents

About the companion website vii

About the companion website

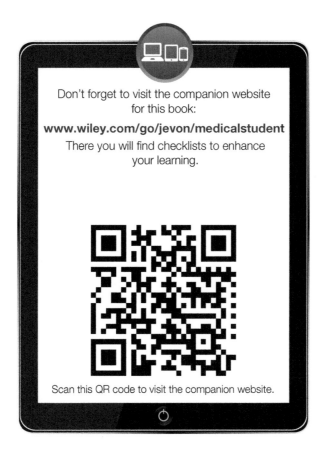

Don't forget to visit the companion website for this book:

www.wiley.com/go/jevon/medicalstudent

There you will find checklists to enhance your learning.

Scan this QR code to visit the companion website.

1 ABCDE: Assessment and treatment of the acutely Ill patient

ABCDE approach: Guiding principles

- Undertake a complete initial ABCDE assessment (Box 1.1); reassess regularly
- Treat life-threatening problems first, before proceeding to the next part of assessment.
- Evaluate the effects of treatment and/or other interventions
- Recognise the circumstances when additional help is required
- Ensure effective communication
- Call for help early (SBAR) (Box 1.2)

Medical Student Survival Skills: The Acutely Ill Patient, First Edition. Philip Jevon, Konnur Ramkumar, and Emma Jenkinson.
© 2020 John Wiley & Sons Ltd. Published 2020 by John Wiley & Sons Ltd.
Companion website: www.wiley.com/go/jevon/medicalstudent

Initial approach

Safety
- Ensure safe approach: check the environment and remove any hazards
- Take measures to minimise the risk of cross infection

Simple question
- Ask the patient a simple question, e.g. 'How are you, sir?' If there is a normal verbal response the patient has a patent airway, is breathing, and has cerebral perfusion. If the patient can only speak in short sentences, they may have extreme respiratory distress, and failure to respond is a clear indicator of serious illness. If there is an inappropriate response or if there is no response, the patient may be acutely ill

> **NB** If the patent is unconscious: summon help from colleagues immediately.

General appearance
- Note the general appearance of the patient, e.g. comfortable or distressed, content or concerned, colour and posture

Vital signs monitoring
- Attach vital signs monitoring, e.g. pulse oximetry, electrocardiogram (ECG) and continuous non-invasive blood pressure (BP) monitoring

Airway

- Patient talking: there is a patent airway
- Complete airway obstruction: there are no breath sounds at the mouth or nose
- Partial airway obstruction: air entry diminished, often noisy breathing

Look
- Look for the signs of airway obstruction, e.g. paradoxical chest and abdominal movements ('see-saw' respirations); central cyanosis is a late sign of airway obstruction

Listen
- Gurgling: fluid in the mouth or upper airway
- Snoring: tongue partially obstructing the pharynx
- Crowing: laryngeal spasm

- Inspiratory stridor: 'croaking respirations' indicating partial upper airway obstruction, e.g. foreign body, laryngeal oedema
- Expiratory wheeze: noisy musical sound caused by turbulent flow of air through narrowed bronchi and bronchioles, more pronounced on expiration; causes include asthma and chronic obstructive pulmonary disease (COPD)

Feel
- Feel for signs of airway obstruction. Place your face or hand in front of the patient's mouth to determine whether there is movement of air

---

OSCE Key Learning Points

Causes of airway obstruction
- ✔ Tongue: commonest cause of airway obstruction in a semi-conscious or unconscious patient – relaxation of the muscles supporting the tongue can result in it falling back and blocking the pharynx
- ✔ Vomit, blood, and secretions
- ✔ Foreign body
- ✔ Tissue swelling: causes include anaphylaxis, trauma, or infection
- ✔ Laryngeal oedema (due to burns, inflammation, or allergy occurring at the level of the larynx)
- ✔ Laryngeal spasm (due to foreign body, airway stimulation, or secretions/blood in the airway)
- ✔ Tracheobronchial obstruction (due to aspiration of gastric contents, secretions, pulmonary oedema fluid, or bronchospasm)

Treatment of airway obstruction
- If airway obstruction is identified, treat appropriately; for example suction, lateral position, and insertion of oropharyngeal airway are often effective
- Administer oxygen 15 l min^{-1} via a non-rebreathe oxygen mask as appropriate
- If necessary, call for help early (SBAR)

Breathing

Inspect
- Look for signs of respiratory distress: tachypnoea, sweating, central cyanosis, use of the accessory muscles of respiration, abdominal breathing, and posture (e.g. pyramid position)

- Count the respiratory rate (normal respiratory rate in adults is approximately 12–20 min^{-1}): tachypnoea is often the first sign that the patient is becoming acutely ill and causes include pneumonia, pulmonary embolism (PE), heart failure, and shock; bradypnoea is an ominous sign and possible causes include drugs, opiates, fatigue, hypothermia, head injury, and central nervous system (CNS) depression

OSCE Key Learning Points

Causes of tachypnoea
- ✔ Respiratory pathology, e.g. acute asthma attack, PE
- ✔ Heart failure
- ✔ Acidosis
- ✔ Normal physiological response, e.g. exercise

OSCE Key Learning Points

Causes of bradypnoea
- ✔ Medications, e.g. opiates
- ✔ Head injury
- ✔ CNS depression
- ✔ Hypothermia

- Assess the depth of breathing. Ascertain whether chest movement is equal on both sides. Unilateral movement of the chest suggests unilateral disease, e.g. pneumothorax, pneumonia, or pleural effusion. Kussmaul's breathing (air hunger) is characterised by deep, rapid respirations due to stimulation of the respiratory centre by metabolic acidosis, e.g. in ketoacidosis and chronic renal failure.
- Assess the pattern (rhythm) of breathing. A Cheyne–Stokes breathing pattern (periods of apnoea alternating with periods of hyperpnoea) can be associated with brainstem ischaemia, cerebral injury, and severe left ventricular failure (altered carbon dioxide sensitivity of the respiratory centre)
- Note the presence of any chest deformity, e.g. kyphosis, as this could increase the risk of deterioration in the patient's ability to breathe normally

- If the patient has a chest drain, check it is patent and functioning effectively
- Note the presence of abdominal distension (could limit diaphragmatic movement, thereby exacerbating respiratory distress)
- Note the oxygen saturation (SaO_2) reading (normal is 94–100%); in a COPD patient normal can be 88–92%
- Check the inspired oxygen concentration (%) being administered to the patient; adjust if necessary

 Common misinterpretations and pitfalls

Pulse oximetry does not detect hypercapnia and that, if the patient is receiving oxygen therapy, the SaO_2 may be normal in the presence of a very high $PaCO_2$.

Palpate
- Check chest expansion
- Palpate the chest wall to detect surgical emphysema or crepitus (suggesting a pneumothorax until proven otherwise)
- Perform chest percussion

OSCE Key Learning Points

Causes of different percussion notes
- ✔ *Resonant*: air-filled lung
- ✔ *Dull*: liver, spleen, heart, lung consolidation/collapse
- ✔ *Stoney dull*: pleural effusion/thickening
- ✔ *Hyper-resonant*: pneumothorax, emphysema
- ✔ *Tympanitic*: gas-filled viscus

- Check the position of the trachea. Place the tip of your index finger into the suprasternal notch, let it slip either side of the trachea and determine whether it fits more easily into one or other side of the trachea; deviation of the trachea to one side indicates mediastinal shift (e.g. pneumothorax, lung fibrosis, pleural fluid)

Auscultate

- Auscultate the chest: assess the depth of breathing and the equality of breath sounds on both sides of the chest. Any additional sounds, e.g. crackles, wheeze, and pleural rubs should be noted. Bronchial breathing indicates lung consolidation; absent or reduced sounds suggest a pneumothorax or pleural fluid

Assessing efficacy of breathing, work of breathing, and adequacy of ventilation

- *Efficacy of breathing*: can be assessed by air entry, chest movement, pulse oximetry, arterial blood gas analysis, and capnography
- *Work of breathing*: can be assessed by respiratory rate and accessory muscle use, e.g. neck and abdominal muscles
- *Adequacy of ventilation*: can be assessed by heart rate, skin colour, and mental status

Causes of compromised breathing

Causes of compromised breathing include:
- Respiratory illness, e.g. asthma, COPD, pneumonia
- Lung pathology, e.g. pneumothorax
- Pulmonary embolism
- Pulmonary oedema
- CNS depression
- Drug-induced respiratory depression

Treatment of compromised breathing

- Position patient appropriately (usually in an upright position)
- Administer oxygen 15 l min^{-1} via a non-rebreathe oxygen mask if required and appropriate
- If possible treat the underlying cause
- If necessary, call for help early (SBAR)

Circulation

NB In most medical and surgical emergencies, if shock is present, treat for hyopvolaemic shock until proven otherwise: administer IV fluid challenge to all patients who have tachycardia and cool peripheries, unless the cause of the circulatory shock is obviously cardiac (cardiogenic shock).

Inspect

- Look at the colour of the hands and fingers. Signs of cardiovascular compromise include cool and pale peripheries
- Measure the capillary refill time (CRT). A prolonged CRT (>2 seconds) could indicate poor peripheral perfusion, although other factors, e.g. cool ambient temperature, poor lighting, and old age can also do this
- Note any other signs suggesting poor cardiac output, e.g. reduced conscious level and, if the patient has a urinary catheter, oliguria (urine volume $<0.5\,ml\,kg^{-1}\,h^{-1}$)
- Examine the patient for signs of external haemorrhage from wounds or drains or evidence of internal haemorrhage. Concealed blood loss can be significant, even if drains are empty

Palpate

- Assess the skin temperature of the patient's limbs to determine whether they are warm or cool, the latter suggesting poor peripheral perfusion
- Palpate peripheral and central pulses. Assess for presence, rate, quality, regularity, and equality; a thready pulse suggests a poor cardiac output, whilst a bounding pulse may indicate sepsis
- Assess the state of the veins: if hypovolaemia is present the veins could be underfilled or collapsed
- Check the BP: a low systolic BP suggests shock. However, even in shock, the BP can still be normal as compensatory mechanisms increase peripheral resistance in response to reduced cardiac output. A low diastolic BP suggests arterial vasodilation (e.g. anaphylaxis or sepsis). A narrowed pulse pressure – i.e. the difference between systolic and diastolic pressures (normal pulse pressure is 35–45 mmHg) – suggests arterial vasoconstriction (e.g. cardiogenic shock or hypovolaemia)

Auscultate

- Auscultate the heart

Monitoring

- Commence ECG monitoring
- Arrange for a 12 lead ECG

Causes of circulatory compromise

Causes of circulatory problems include:

- Acute coronary syndrome
- Cardiac arrhythmias
- Shock, e.g. hypovolaemia, septic and anaphylactic shock

- Heart failure
- Pulmonary embolism

Treatment of circulatory compromise
- The specific treatment required for circulatory compromise will depend on the cause; fluid replacement, haemorrhage control, and restoration of tissue perfusion will usually be necessary

Acute coronary syndromes (Box 1.3)

Box 1.3 Acute coronary syndromes

- Unstable angina
- Non-ST-segment-elevation myocardial infarction (NSTEMI)
- ST-segment-elevation myocardial infarction (STEMI)

- If necessary, call for help early (SBAR)
- Assist patient into a comfortable position (usually semi-recumbent position)
- Commence oxygen saturation monitoring and if necessary administer oxygen to achieve an arterial blood oxygen saturation of 94–98% (88–92% in COPD patients)
- Administer aspirin 300 mg orally crushed or chewed (if no known allergy to aspirin)
- Administer glyceryl trinitrate (GTN) sublingually
- Administer analgesia, e.g. morphine (diamorphine) IV and titrate to control symptoms (avoid sedation and respiratory depression)
- Consider the need for an antiemetic
- Consider reperfusion therapy, e.g. percutaneous coronary intervention (For further information see Chapter 13)

Hypovolaemic shock
- Assist patient into a comfortable position (usually supine)
- Ensure open airway and administer oxygen 15 l via a non-rebreathe mask
- Insert a large bore cannula (12–14 G) and commence IV fluid challenge (500 ml stat) (a second large bore cannula may be required)
- Regularly (every 5 minutes) reassess the patient; repeat the fluid challenge if there is no improvement
- If there are symptoms of heart failure (dyspnoea, increased heart rate, raised jugular venous pressure, pulmonary crackles on chest auscultation,

and/or third heart sound) develop, reduce, or stop IV fluid therapy. Seek expert advice concerning alternative treatments to improve tissue perfusion, e.g. inotropes or vasopressors
- Call for help early (SBAR)
- If possible, identify and treat the underlying cause
  (For further information see Chapter 10)

OSCE Key Learning Points

Rapid fluid challenge (over 5–10 minutes)

✔ *Normtensive*: 500 ml of warmed crystalloid, e.g. Hartmann's solution or 0.9% sodium chloride

✔ *Hypotensive*: 1000 ml of warmed crystalloid, e.g. Hartmann's solution or 0.9% sodium chloride

✔ *Known cardiac failure*: 250 ml of warmed crystalloid, e.g. Hartmann's solution or 0.9% sodium chloride and closely monitor patient (auscultate chest for crackles and consider central venous pressure (CVP) line

---

Disability

- Evaluate CNS function
- Undertake a rapid assessment of the patient's level of conscious using AVPU (Box 1.4) and, if necessary (e.g. head injury), the Glasgow coma score (GCS)

Box 1.4 AVPU assessment of level of consciousness

A	Alert
V	Voice (responds to)
P	Pain (responds to)
U	Unresponsive

- Review ABC to exclude hypoxaemia and hypotension
- Check the patient's drug chart for reversible drug-induced causes of altered conscious level

- Undertake bedside glucose measurement to exclude hypoglycaemia
- Examine the pupils (size, equality, reaction to light, and consensual reaction)

NB Altered level of consciousness is the most common underlying cause of a compromised airway in the healthcare setting.

Causes of altered conscious level
Causes of altered conscious level include:
- Severe hypoxia
- Poor cerebral perfusion
- Drugs, e.g. sedatives, opiates
- Cerebral pathology
- Hypercapnia
- Hypoglycaemia
- Alcohol

Treatment of altered conscious level
- Undertake ABC assessment (as earlier in chapter) and exclude or treat hypoxia and hypotension
- If drug-induced altered conscious level is suspected and the effects are reversible, consider an antidote, e.g. naloxone, which can be used with caution for opiate toxicity
- Administer glucose if hypoglycaemia is suspected or confirmed
- Ensure the patient's airway is maintained: consider placing the patient in the lateral (recovery) position
- If necessary, call for help early (SBAR)

Exposure

- Fully expose the patient and undertake a thorough examination and ensure important details are not missed
- In particular, examine the part of the body which is most likely contributing to the patient's ill status, e.g. in suspected anaphylaxis, examine the skin for urticaria
- Maintain the patient's dignity and minimise heat loss
In addition:
- Undertake a full clinical history

- Review the patient's case notes, observations chart, and medications chart
- Study the recorded vital signs: trends are more significant than one-off recordings
- Ensure that prescribed medications are being administered
- Review the results of laboratory, ECG, and radiological investigations
- Consider the level of care the patient requires (e.g. ward, high dependency unit, intensive care unit)
- Record in the patient's case notes any details of assessment, treatment, and response to treatment
- Call for senior help if necessary (SBAR)

OSCE Key Learning Points

Minimising the risk of cross infection

✔ Decontaminate hands with an alcohol-based handrub between caring for different patients and between different care activities for the same patient

✔ If hands are visibly soiled, or potentially grossly contaminated with dirt or organic material, wash with liquid soap and water

✔ Before regular hand decontamination begins, all wrist and ideally hand jewellery should be removed

✔ Cover cuts and abrasions with waterproof dressings

✔ Ensure fingernails are kept short, clean, and free from nail polish

② Management of tachypnoea

> **Definition:** Respiratory rate $> 20\,min^{-1}$.

 NB Tachypnoea is often the first adverse sign seen in acute illness (Box 2.1).

Box 2.1 Clinical signs of acute illness

- Tachypnoea
- Tachycardia
- Hypotension
- Altered level of consciousness (e.g. lethargy, confusion, restlessness, or falling level of consciousness)

Causes

- Asthma
- Heart failure
- Pulmonary embolism
- Pneumonia
- Acute respiratory distress syndrome
- Anaphylaxis
- Shock
- Pneumothorax

Medical Student Survival Skills: The Acutely Ill Patient, First Edition. Philip Jevon,
Konnur Ramkumar, and Emma Jenkinson.
© 2020 John Wiley & Sons Ltd. Published 2020 by John Wiley & Sons Ltd.
Companion website: www.wiley.com/go/jevon/medicalstudent

Other causes include:
- Pain
- Pyrexia
- Exercise

Control of respirations

- Respirations are controlled by the respiratory centre in the medulla oblongata
- Chemoreceptors increase the respiratory rate/depth in response to hypercapnia, hypoxaemia, or acidosis
- In patients with chronic respiratory disease, the respiratory drive is hypoxia (hypoxic drive)

Identification of underlying factors to respiratory disease

- Smoking – if so, how many cigarettes per day
- Orthopnoea – the need to sleep in an upright position propped up with pillows suggests a cardiac cause to breathless
- Does the patient live in a damp home
- Occupation: in a furnace or building trade using asbestos
- Recent foreign holiday or trip – tuberculosis
- Sputum – blood-stained or purulent

Association with acute illness

- Most common clinical abnormality found in critical illness
- Important indicator of an at-risk patient
- A raised respiratory rate ($>27\,min^{-1}$) occurs in 54% of patients in the 72 hours preceding cardiac arrest
- Abnormal respiratory rate values indicate that patients have a higher mortality risk: a 90 day mortality of 20% compared with 1.6% overall

Assessment of breathing

NB During the assessment of breathing, it is important to quickly diagnose and treat any life-threatening breathing problems, e.g. acute asthma.

- Environment around bed: oxygen, inhalers, nebuliser, sputum pots, chest drain
- Patient's general appearance: a breathless patient usually looks anxious
- Patient's colour: central cyanosis is usually a severe adverse sign
- Patient's posture: sitting upright, 'pyramid position', or leaning forward resting on a bedside table may indicate dyspnoea
- Talk to the patient: a breathless patient may have difficulty talking, e.g. being unable to complete a sentence in one breath is considered a severe adverse sign during an asthma attack
- Respiratory rate: normal range 12–20 min^{-1}
- Mechanics of breathing: unilateral chest movement indicates lung pathology causes of which include pneumothorax, pneumonia, and collapsed lung
- Depth of breathing: deep breathing may be observed if the patient is having a panic attack
- Oxygen saturation (SaO_2) reading: the normal reading is usually 94–100%
- Chest palpation: symmetry and expansion
- Chest percussion
- Trachea: central or deviated
- Chest auscultation
- Signs of partial airway obstruction (Box 2.2)
- Arterial blood gas analysis (if indicated)

Box 2.2 Signs of partial airway obstruction

- Wheeze (lower airway)
- Stridor (upper airway)
- Gurgling (fluid in upper airway)

OSCE Key Learning Points

Counting respiratory rate

✔ Be discrete to ensure accuracy, e.g. 'check pulse' for 1 minute and during this minute count the respiratory rate.

Management of tachypnoea

- ABCDE
- Request appropriate monitoring, e.g. pulse oximetry
- Ensure the patient has a clear airway

- Assist the patient into a comfortable position: usually sitting up, propped up with pillows. Sometimes sitting on the edge of the bed with feet touching the floor will be helpful
- Administer oxygen if necessary
- Identify and where possible treat the underlying cause
- Secure IV access; appropriate bloods
- Request appropriate investigations, e.g. chest X-ray, arterial blood gases
- Repeat ABCDE: assess and reassess effectiveness of interventions/ treatment
- Request senior help if necessary: SBAR

 Common misinterpretations and pitfalls

Managing patients who are breathless in the supine position: if possible sit them up particularly in heart failure.

3 Management of bradycardia

Definition: Heart rate <60 min⁻¹.

Causes

- Physiological, e.g. fit person
- Cardiac origin, e.g. ischaemia, atrioventricular (AV) block
- Non-cardiac origin, e.g. hypoxia, electrolyte abnormality, hypothermia, and cerebral bleed
- Medications, e.g. beta-adrenoreceptor blockers, digoxin, and amiodarone

NB Bradycardia will be a normal finding in some patients, particularly in those who are young and fit; it can also be associated with beta-adrenoreceptor blocker therapy.

ECG examples of bradycardias

- Sinus bradycardia (Figure 3.1)
- Second degree heart block type I (Figure 3.2)
- Second degree heart block type II (Figure 3.3)
- Third degree (complete) heart block (Figure 3.4)

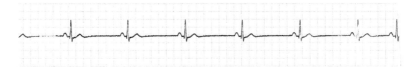

Figure 3.1 Sinus bradycardia.

Medical Student Survival Skills: The Acutely Ill Patient, First Edition. Philip Jevon, Konnur Ramkumar, and Emma Jenkinson.
© 2020 John Wiley & Sons Ltd. Published 2020 by John Wiley & Sons Ltd.
Companion website: www.wiley.com/go/jevon/medicalstudent

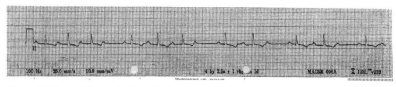

Figure 3.2 Second degree AV block Mobitz type I.

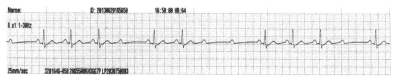

Figure 3.3 Second degree AV block Mobitz type II.

(a)

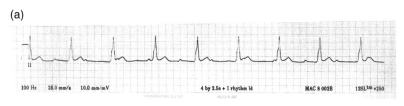

(b)

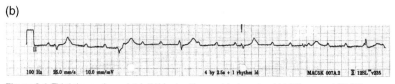

Figure 3.4 Third degree (complete) AV block with a ventricular rate of (a) 50 bpm and (b) 35 bpm.

Indications for treatment

The emergency treatment of bradycardia will depend upon two important clinical factors:

- The presence of certain adverse clinical features (Box 3.1): these will determine whether treatment is indicated and the urgency with which it is required
- The risk of asystole (Box 3.2)

Box 3.1 Bradycardia: Adverse clinical features

- *Circulatory shock*: hypotension (systolic blood pressure [BP] <90 mmHg), pallor, sweating, cold and clammy extremities (increased sympathetic activity), and impaired level of consciousness (e.g. drowsiness and confusion) due to reduced cerebral blood flow

- *Syncope*: transient loss of consciousness due to reduced cerebral perfusion
- *Heart failure*: shortness of breath, pulmonary crackles on auscultation, and pulmonary oedema on chest X-ray; peripheral oedema, raised jugular venous pressure, and hepatic engorgement
- *Myocardial ischaemia*: chest pain and/or ST ischaemic changes on a 12 lead electrocardiogram (ECG); these indicate that the cardiac arrhythmia is causing myocardial ischaemia (particular significant if the patient has existing coronary artery disease or structural heart disease, because it could cause further life-threatening complications including cardiopulmonary arrest)
- *Extreme bradycardia* (typically heart rate ≤40): although this is usually defined as a heart rate <40 beats per minute (bpm), higher rates may not be well tolerated by some patients with poor cardiac reserve

Box 3.2 Bradycardia: Risk of asystole

- Recent asystole (Figure 3.5)
- Second degree AV block type II
- Complete heart block with wide QRS complex
- Ventricular pause >3 seconds

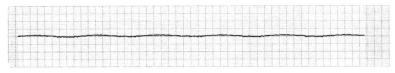

Figure 3.5 Asystole.

Principles of the use of the adult bradycardia algorithm

- The Resuscitation Council (UK)'s adult bradycardia algorithm (Figure 3.6) is designed for non-specialists in order to provide effective and safe treatment in the emergency situation
- If the patient is not acutely ill, other treatment options may be considered and there is usually time to seek help from a senior clinician, e.g. cardiologist

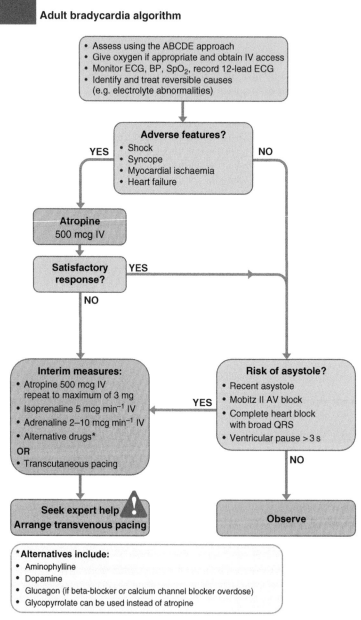

Figure 3.6 Resuscitation Council (UK) adult bradycardia algorithm.

- The algorithm is specifically designed for the emergency situation and is not intended to encompass all clinical situations
- Arrows indicate progression from one stage of treatment to the next, but only if the cardiac arrhythmia persists
- Several variables will influence the treatment including the cardiac arrhythmia, the haemodynamic status of the patient, local procedures, and local circumstances/facilities/expertise
- Drug doses are based on average body weight; in some situations adjustments to the dose may be required
- Expert help must be summoned early if necessary

OSCE Key Learning Points

Common causes of bradycardia

✔ Beta-adreno-receptor blockers
✔ Cardiac ischaemia
✔ Bradycardia will be a normal finding in some patients

Treatment of bradycardia

- ABCDE approach
- Consider lying the patient flat and raising their legs (if low BP)
- If necessary, administer high concentration oxygen and commence pulse oximetry
- Try to ascertain the cause of the bradycardia and treat if reversible
- Secure IV access and commence ECG monitoring; establish that the patient has bradycardia
- Record an ECG rhythm strip and 12 lead ECG if necessary
- If the patient is hypotensive and is feeling light-headed, lie flat and raise their legs
- If adverse clinical features are present (e.g. systolic BP <90 mmHg, heart rate <40 bpm, altered conscious level, heart failure) administer atropine 500 µg IV and repeat every 3–5 minutes up to a maximum of 3 mg IV if necessary. Care should be taken in patients with an acute coronary syndrome because the increase in heart rate could worsen the ischaemia
- If the response to atropine is unsatisfactory, consider transcutaneous pacing; in some clinical situations it may be more appropriate to try second line pharmacological treatment (Box 3.3) first

NB The dose of atropine should not be <500 µg as this may cause paradoxical slowing of the heart rate.

Box 3.3 Second line pharmaceutical treatment for bradycardia

- Consider using glucagon IV when a beta-blocker or calcium channel blocker is the probable cause of the bradycardia
- Consider digoxin-specific antibody fragments when digoxin toxicity is the probable cause of the bradycardia
- Consider theophylline 100–200 mg IV when bradycardia complicates inferior myocardial infarction, spinal cord injury, or cardiac transplantation

---

 NB Do not administer atropine to a patient with a heart transplant – the heart is denervated and will not respond to vagal blockade by atropine, which could result in paradoxical sinus arrest or high grade AV block.

- If there is no response to atropine and the patient remains unstable and/or there is a risk of asystole (Box 3.2), ensure that appropriate help, e.g. a cardiologist, has been requested because pacing will usually be required. The definitive treatment will be transvenous pacing, but while awaiting the appropriate expertise and facilities to be arranged, interim measures to help prevent deterioration and improve the patient's condition include transcutaneous (external) pacing or fist pacing if this is not available, or an adrenaline or isoprenaline infusion

---

OSCE Key Learning Points

Initial management of bradycardia

✔ ABCDE – oxygen, IV access, and atropine if necessary

Transcutaneous (external) pacing

- Cardiac pacing is the delivery of a low electric current to the heart to stimulate myocardial contraction
- Transcutaneous (external) pacing is quick and easily established and buys time for the spontaneous recovery of the conduction system or for more definitive treatment to be established, e.g. transvenous pacing
- Transcutaneous pacing can be painful: analgesia and sedation may be required

Procedure
- If appropriate, explain the procedure to the patient
- Ideally, first remove excess chest hair from the pacing electrode sites by clipping close to the patient's skin using a pair of scissors
- Attach the pacing electrodes following the manufacturer's instructions.
- *Pacing-only electrodes*: attach the anterior electrode on the left anterior chest, midway between the xiphoid process and the left nipple (V2–V3 ECG electrode position) and attach the posterior electrode below the left scapula, lateral to the spine and at the same level as the anterior electrode – this anterior/posterior configuration will ensure that the position of the electrodes does not interfere with defibrillation. ECG monitoring will usually need to be established if an older pacing system is used
- *Multifunctional electrodes* (pacing and defibrillation): place the anterior electrode below the right clavicle and the lateral electrode in the mid-axillary line lateral to the left nipple (V6 ECG electrode position) – this anterior/lateral position is convenient during cardiopulmonary resuscitation (CPR) as chest compressions do not have to be interrupted
- Check that the pacing electrodes and connecting cables are applied following the manufacturer's recommendations; if they are reversed pacing may be ineffective or high capture thresholds may be required
- Adjust the ECG gain (size) accordingly. This will help ensure that the intrinsic QRS complexes are sensed
- Select demand mode on the pacing unit on the defibrillator
- Select an appropriate rate for external pacing, usually 60–90 min^{-1}
- Set the pacing current at the lowest level, turn on the pacemaker unit and while observing both the patient and the ECG, gradually increase the current until electrical capture occurs (QRS complexes following the pacing spike). Electrical capture usually occurs when the current delivered is in the range of 50–100 mA

- Check pulse: palpable pulse = mechanical capture
- Request expert help and prepare for transvenous pacing. If there is no pulse, start CPR. If there is good electrical capture, but no mechanical capture, this is indicative of a non-viable myocardium

 NB There is no electrical hazard if in contact with the patient during transcutaneous pacing.

4 Management of sinus tachycardia

Sinus tachycardia (Figure 4.1) is a common finding in the critically ill patient. It is not classed as a tachyarrhythmia; it is usually a response to another physiological or pathological state.

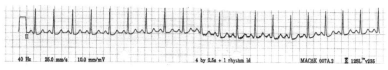

40 Hz   25.0 mm/s   10.0 mm/mV   4 by 2.5s + 1 rhythm ld   MAC5K 007A.2   Σ 12SL™v235

Figure 4.1 Example of sinus tachycardia.

Causes

Causes include:
- Hypovolaemia
- Sepsis
- Heart failure
- Myocardial infarction
- Severe pain
- Anxiety
- Thyrotoxicosis
- Medications, e.g. beta II agonists (e.g. salbutamol)
- Toxicity, (e.g. SSRI overdose or cocaine use)

ECG features

- Heart rate is > 100 but generally < 140 bpm
- Usually regular
- P waves present; P waves associated with QRS complexes
- Non-paroxysmal, i.e. it does not start and end abruptly – a common feature of tachyarrhythmias

Medical Student Survival Skills: The Acutely Ill Patient, First Edition. Philip Jevon, Konnur Ramkumar, and Emma Jenkinson.
© 2020 John Wiley & Sons Ltd. Published 2020 by John Wiley & Sons Ltd.
Companion website: www.wiley.com/go/jevon/medicalstudent

Common misinterpretations and pitfalls

An atrial flutter with a 2 : 1 atrioventricular (AV) block can mimic sinus tachycardia. The ventricular rate is typically 150 bpm and constant.

Treatment of sinus tachycardia

- ABCDE
- Direct treatment to treat the underlying cause, not the sinus tachycardia

OSCE Key Learning Points

Management of sinus tachycardia

✔ Identify and treat the underlying cause

5 Management of other tachycardias

OSCE Key Learning Points

Management of sinus tachycardia

✔ Identify and treat the underlying cause (see Chapter 4)

Causes

- Physiological: e.g. stress
- Cardiac origin: e.g. ischaemia, valve disease, cardiomyopathy
- Non-cardiac origin: e.g. hypoxia, electrolyte abnormality, hypothermia, cerebral bleed
- Medications: e.g. anti-arrhythmic medications (e.g. amiodarone)

ECG examples of tachycardias

- Atrial fibrillation (Figure 5.1)
- Narrow complex tachycardia (Figure 5.2)
- Broad complex tachycardia (Figure 5.3)

Medical Student Survival Skills: The Acutely Ill Patient, First Edition. Philip Jevon, Konnur Ramkumar, and Emma Jenkinson.
© 2020 John Wiley & Sons Ltd. Published 2020 by John Wiley & Sons Ltd.
Companion website: www.wiley.com/go/jevon/medicalstudent

(a)

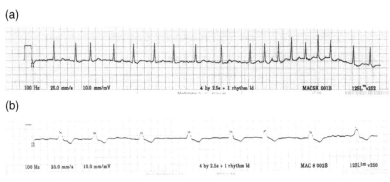

(b)

Figure 5.1 (a and b) Atrial fibrillation.

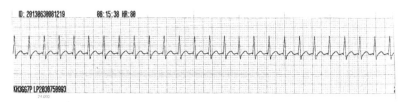

Figure 5.2 Junctional tachycardia.

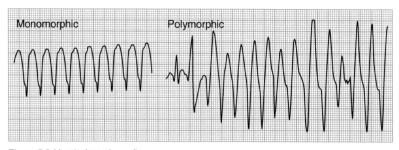

Figure 5.3 Ventricular tachycardia.

OSCE Key Learning Points

✔ A broad complex tachycardia is normally ventricular in origin (ventricular tachycardia)

Indications for treatment

The emergency treatment of tachycardia will depend upon three important clinical factors:

- The presence of certain adverse clinical features (Box 5.1): these will determine whether treatment is indicated and the urgency with which it is required
- Whether it is narrow QRS complex or broad QRS complex tachycardia
- Whether the QRS rhythm is regular or irregular (latter probably atrial fibrillation)

Box 5.1 Tachycardia: Adverse clinical features

- *Circulatory shock*: hypotension (systolic blood pressure [BP] <90 mmHg), pallor, sweating, cold and clammy extremities (increased sympathetic activity), and impaired level of consciousness (e.g. drowsiness and confusion) due to reduced cerebral blood flow
- *Syncope*: transient loss of consciousness due to reduced cerebral perfusion
- *Heart failure*: shortness of breath, pulmonary crackles on auscultation, and pulmonary oedema on chest X-ray; peripheral oedema, raised jugular venous pressure, and hepatic engorgement
- *Myocardial ischaemia*: chest pain and/or ST ischaemic changes on a 12 lead electrocardiogram (ECG); these indicate that the cardiac arrhythmia is causing myocardial ischaemia (this is particular significant if the patient has existing coronary artery disease or structural heart disease, because it could cause further life-threatening complications including cardiopulmonary arrest)

Principles of using the adult tachycardia (with pulse) algorithm

- The Resuscitation Council (UK)'s adult tachycardia (with pulse) algorithm (Figure 5.4) is designed for non-specialists in order to provide effective and safe treatment in the emergency situation
- If the patient is not acutely ill, other treatment options may be considered and there is usually time to seek help from a senior clinician, e.g. cardiologist
- The algorithm is specifically designed for the emergency situation and is not intended to encompass all clinical situations

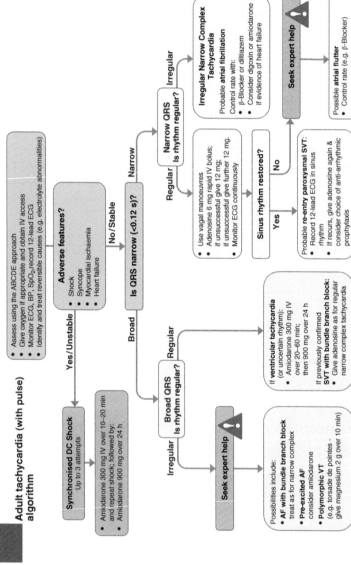

2010 Resuscitation Guidelines

Adult tachycardia (with pulse) algorithm

Resuscitation Council (UK)

- Assess using the ABCDE approach
- Give oxygen if appropriate and obtain IV access
- Monitor ECG, BP, SpO$_2$, record 12-lead ECG
- Identify and treat reversible causes (e.g. electrolyte abnormalities)

Adverse features?
- Shock
- Syncope
- Myocardial ischaemia
- Heart failure

Yes/Unstable

Synchronised DC Shock
Up to 3 attempts

- Amiodarone 300 mg IV over 10–20 min and repeat shock; followed by:
- Amiodarone 900 mg over 24 h

No/Stable

Is QRS narrow (<0.12 s)?

Broad

Narrow

Broad QRS
Is rhythm regular?

Irregular

Seek expert help ⚠

Possibilities include:
- **AF with bundle branch block** treat as for narrow complex
- **Pre-excited AF** consider amiodarone
- **Polymorphic VT** (e.g. torsade de pointes - give magnesium 2 g over 10 min)

Regular

If ventricular tachycardia (or uncertain rhythm):
- Amiodarone 300 mg IV over 20–60 min; then 900 mg over 24 h

If previously confirmed **SVT with bundle branch block:**
- Give adenosine as for regular narrow complex tachycardia

Narrow QRS
Is rhythm regular?

Regular

- Use vagal manoeuvres
- Adenosine 6 mg rapid IV bolus; if unsuccessful give 12 mg; if unsuccessful give further 12 mg.
- Monitor ECG continuously

Sinus rhythm restored?

Yes

Probable re-entry paroxysmal SVT:
- Record 12-lead ECG in sinus rhythm
- If recurs, give adenosine again & consider choice of anti-arrhythmic prophylaxis

No

Seek expert help ⚠

Possible **atrial flutter**
- Control rate (e.g. β-Blocker)

Irregular

Irregular Narrow Complex Tachycardia
Probable **atrial fibrillation**
Control rate with:
- β-Blocker or diltiazem
- Consider digoxin or amiodarone if evidence of heart failure

Figure 5.4 Resuscitation Council (UK) Adult tachycardia (with pulse) algorithm.

- Arrows indicate progression from one stage of treatment to the next, but only if the cardiac arrhythmia persists
- Several variables will influence the treatment including the cardiac arrhythmia, the haemodynamic status of the patient, local procedures, and local circumstances/facilities/expertise
- Drug doses are based on average body weight; in some situations adjustments to the dose may be required
- Expert help must be summoned early if necessary

NB The adult tachycardia (with pulse) algorithm is not suitable for sinus tachycardia.

OSCE Key Learning Points

Common causes of tachycardia
- ✔ Cardiac ischaemia
- ✔ Electrolyte imbalance
- ✔ Medications

Treatment of tachycardia

The Resuscitation Council (UK) tachycardia (with pulse) algorithm (Figure 5.4) works on the basis that, irrespective of the exact underlying ECG rhythm, most of the initial treatment principles for a tachyarrhythmia are the same.

- ABCDE to assess for adverse clinical features (Box 5.1)
- While undertaking this assessment, ensure high concentration oxygen is commenced, appropriate monitoring is established (oxygen saturation and ECG), and IV access is secured
- Establish that the patient has a tachycardia, taking care to ensure that it is not sinus tachycardia (see Chapter 4)
- If the patient is hypotensive or is feeling lightheaded, lie them flat
- Ensure appropriate help is called
- Record a single lead ECG strip from the monitor
- If possible record a 12 lead ECG; this will help to establish the correct interpretation of the rhythm, either before treatment or retrospectively if necessary with the help of an expert

- Identify and treat any underlying causes, e.g. electrolyte abnormalities, particularly hypokalaemia
- If the patient is unstable (e.g. altered conscious level, systolic BP < 90 mmHg, chest pain, heart failure), prepare for synchronised electrical cardioversion (see later in this chapter)
- If the patient is stable, treatment will depend on whether the rhythm is regular or irregular and whether the QRS complex is narrow (< 0.12 seconds or 3 small squares) or broad (0.12 seconds or more); treatment options initially include vagal manoeuvres and anti-arrhythmic drugs
- Once the arrhythmia has been successfully treated, repeat the 12 lead ECG to enable detection of any underlying abnormalities that may require long-term therapy

Vagal manoeuvres

- Used to stimulate the vagus nerve and induce a reflex slowing of the heart
- Successful in terminating 25% of narrow complex tachycardias
- *Carotid sinus massage*: this should not be used in the presence of a carotid bruit as atheromatous plaque rupture could embolise into the cerebral circulation causing a cerebral vascular accident; elderly patients are more vulnerable to plaque rupture and cerebral vascular complications. Therefore it should only be undertaken by an expert practitioner
- *Valsalva manoeuvre*: this is a forced expiration against a closed glottis, e.g. ask the patient to blow into a 20 ml syringe with enough force to push the plunger back

Anti-arrhythmic drugs

As anti-arrhythmic drug therapy has a slower onset of action and is less reliable than electrical cardioversion in converting a tachycardia to a normal sinus rhythm, drugs are generally reserved for stable patients without adverse signs. Electrical cardioversion is used in unstable patients displaying adverse signs.

NB All anti-arrhythmic treatments can be pro-arrhythmic, i.e. clinical deterioration of the patient may due to the treatment rather than lack of effect.

Adenosine
- Very effective at terminating tachyarrhythmias that originate in the atrioventricular (AV) junction
- Very short half-life (10–15 seconds)
- Administered as a rapid IV bolus followed by a flush
- Recommended initial dose is 6 mg IV, two further doses of 12 mg may be administered if required
- Side effects include bronchospasm, AV heart block, flushing, and chest pain
- During administration, continuous ECG monitoring is required

Digoxin
- Commonly used for atrial fibrillation, particular in the presence of heart failure
- Emergency loading dose: 0.75–1 mg IV over at least 2 hours
- Maintenance dose is 125–250 µg daily taken orally
- Renal function and digoxin plasma levels should be closely monitored

Amiodarone
- Widely used for the management of tachyarrhythmias
- Standard dose is 300 mg IV over 10–60 minutes (depending on the circumstances and haemodynamic stability of the patient) followed by an infusion of 900 mg over 24 hours
- Cannot be mixed with normal saline (5% dextrose is usually used as a diluting solution)
- Adverse side effects include hypotension, bradycardia, and thrombophlebitis (central vein preferred for IV administration)

Verapamil
- Occasionally used for narrow complex tachycardia
- Initial dose is 2.5–5 mg IV over 2 minutes; repeated doses may be necessary

Synchronised electrical cardioversion

- This is the synchronised delivery of a shock to the myocardium to terminate a tachyarrhythmia
- It is indicated if the patient has a tachycardia, is unstable, and adverse signs are present (Figure 5.4) (it can also be considered if chemical or drug therapy is ineffective)

- Shock must be delivered on the R wave not the T wave, as the delivery of the shock during the refractory period of the cardiac cycle (T wave) could induce ventricular fibrillation. The defibrillator must therefore be synchronised with the patient's ECG

Shock energies

- *Broad complex tachycardia and atrial fibrillation*: 120–150 J biphasic (200 J monophasic) is recommended initially
- *Regular narrow complex tachycardia or atrial flutter*: 70–120 J biphasic (100 J monophasic) is recommended initially

NB Due to the risk of a cerebral embolism arising from stasis of blood in the left atrium, a patient with atrial fibrillation >48 hours should normally not receive electrical synchronised cardioversion until they have been fully anticoagulated or transoesophageal echocardiography has confirmed the absence of an atrial clot.

Procedure

- If possible record a 12 lead ECG
- Explain the procedure to the patient. Consent should be obtained if possible. If the patient is conscious, they must be anaesthetised or sedated for the procedure (anaesthetist should ideally be present)
- Ensure resuscitation equipment is immediately at hand
- Establish ECG monitoring using the defibrillator that is going to be used for cardioversion
- Select a monitoring lead that provides a clear ECG trace on the monitor, e.g. lead II
- Press the 'synch' button on the defibrillator
- Check the ECG trace to ensure that only the R waves are being synchronised; i.e. a 'synchronised dot or arrow' should appear on each R wave and not on any other parts of the ECG complex such as tall T waves
- Apply defibrillation gel pads to the patient's chest, one just to the right of the sternum, below the right clavicle, and the other in the mid-axillary line, approximately level with the V6 ECG electrode or female breast
- Select the appropriate energy level on the defibrillator
- Place the defibrillator paddles firmly on the defibrillation pads. It is not necessary to apply the paddles according to their namesakes, i.e. sternum to sternum and apex to apex

- Perform a visual sweep to ensure that all personnel are clear and that the oxygen has been removed
- Charge the defibrillator and shout 'Stand clear'
- Check the ECG monitor to ensure that the patient is still in the tachyarrhythmia that requires cardioversion, that the synchronised button is still activated, and that it is still synchronising with the R waves
- Press both discharge buttons simultaneously to discharge the shock. There is usually a slight delay between pressing the shock buttons and shock discharge
- Reassess the ECG trace. The 'synch' button will usually need to be reactivated if further cardioversion is required (on some defibrillators it is necessary to actually switch off the 'synch' button if further cardioversion is not indicated). Stepwise increases in energy will be required if cardioversion needs to be repeated. Amiodarone is indicated if three attempts at cardioversion have been unsuccessful
- Record a post successful cardioversion 12 lead ECG
- Monitor the patient's vital signs until there is full recovery from the anaesthetic or sedative
- Ensure accurate documentation of the procedure

OSCE Key Learning Points

Initial management of tachycardia

✔ ABCDE – oxygen, IV access, and record 12 lead ECG

Management of oliguria

> **Definition:** Production of abnormally small amounts of urine (between 100 and 400 ml per 24 hours).

Background

- Can be a sign that the patient is sick and is deteriorating
- Usually associated with hypovolaemia caused by restricted fluid intake or excessive fluid loss
- Timely appropriate intervention may re-establish urine output and protect renal function – this could prevent further deterioration and progression to acute renal failure, a life-threatening condition that is becoming increasingly common in critically ill patients

NB Fluid balance is essential for the normal functioning of all the systems in the body because it helps to maintain body temperature and cell shape, and assists in the transportation of nutrients, gases, and waste products.

Monitoring fluid balance

- Monitoring fluid balance is important, particularly in the critically ill patient
- Many factors can affect fluid status including physiological mechanisms, disease processes, and side effects of treatment
- Fluid input and output (oral intake, urine output, wound and nasogastric drainage, and all drug and fluid infusions) should be closely monitored following local early warning score (EWS) protocols (usually at least hourly)

Medical Student Survival Skills: The Acutely Ill Patient, First Edition. Philip Jevon, Konnur Ramkumar, and Emma Jenkinson.
© 2020 John Wiley & Sons Ltd. Published 2020 by John Wiley & Sons Ltd.
Companion website: www.wiley.com/go/jevon/medicalstudent

Prerequisites for normal urine output

Prerequisites for normal urine output include:
- Adequate renal perfusion – renal blood flow remains constant if the mean blood pressure is between 70 and 170 mmHg
- Normal renal function
- No obstruction to the flow of urine

Definitions of abnormal urine output

- *Oliguria*: 100–400 ml in 24 hours
- *Anuria*: < 100 ml in 24 hours
- *Absolute anuria*: 0 ml in 24 hours

 Common misinterpretations and pitfalls

Absolute anuria is rare and is usually associated with a blocked urinary catheter.

Causes

Causes of include:
- Pre-renal, e.g. hypovolaemia, hypotension
- Renal, e.g. acute tubular necrosis
- Post-renal, e.g. ureteric stone, retention of urine

Fluid challenge

- The aim of a fluid challenge is to produce a significant and rapid increase in plasma volume, which will hopefully then stabilise the patient's condition. This will buy time so that expert help can be sought and a more definite diagnosis made
- A fluid challenge (usually 500 ml of a crystalloid, e.g. 0.9% normal saline) is administered over approximately 15 minutes; the patient is then closely monitored for signs of improvement, e.g. decreased respiratory and pulse rates, a rise in blood pressure and improved level of consciousness. The fluid bolus may need to be repeated

OSCE Key Learning Points

✔ Isotonic crystalloid, e.g. 0.9% normal saline, is the preferred choice of fluid

✔ Fluids containing dextrose are not used for initial resuscitation because they rapidly distribute throughout both the intracellular and extracellular fluid compartments in the body, with very little remaining in the circulation

Treatment of oliguria

- ABCDE approach
- Administer high-flow oxygen if required
- If the patient is hypotensive, ideally position them in a supine position
- If the patient has a urinary catheter, ensure that oliguria is not due to a mechanical problem, e.g. blocked catheter, kinked catheter tubing
- Exclude retention of urine as the cause of oliguria. Opiates can cause retention of urine by affecting bladder sphincter control and removing the sensation of a full bladder (more common in men especially if there are existing symptoms of prostatism)
- Secure IV access and, if necessary, administer a fluid challenge as prescribed, monitoring its effect. It may be necessary to repeat the fluid challenge
- If the patient does not have a urinary catheter in situ, insert one
- Attempt to establish the cause of the oliguria. Perform urinalysis and send off a urine sample for microscopy, culture, and sensitivity MC&S)
- Ensure appropriate laboratory investigations are ordered, e.g. regular measurement of serum sodium, potassium, urea, and creatinine; 24 hour urine volume may be required to assess fluid and electrolyte balance
- Closely monitor the patient's fluid balance charts from the preceding few days and compare the corresponding serum and urine urea and electrolyte results. This will help evaluate the patient's response to fluid administration and will guide the fluid regime over the next 12–24 hours
- Regularly monitor the patient's fluid balance in combination with vital signs monitoring

- Consider reviewing the use of nephrotoxic drugs, e.g. non-steroidal anti-inflammatory drugs (NSAIDs), frusemide, gentamicin, and ciclosporin, as these may need to be omitted

 Common misinterpretations and pitfalls

Diuretic therapy may need to be omitted because it can be ineffective in preventing and treating acute renal failure.

7 Management of pyrexia

Definitions:
- *Pyrexia* is an elevation of body temperature above the normal daily variation
- *Hyperpyrexia* is a temperature >40 °C
- *Fever* is an abnormal rise in body temperature, usually accompanied by shivering, headache, and, if severe, delirium
- *Hyperthermia* is a body temperature greatly above normal
- *Malignant hyperthermia* is a rapid rise of temperature to a dangerous level (usually 41–45 °C)

Background

- Pyrexia is abnormal, an adverse sign, and an important component of early warning scoring systems and can be associated with serious life-threatening illness
- Management is dictated by the severity of the pyrexia and its probable cause, the patient's condition, prognosis, local protocols, and, of course, whether the patient is symptomatic, e.g. feeling hot, sweating profusely, etc.
- It is a common clinical finding in acute illness
- A sudden rise in temperature usually indicates infection, although there are many other non-infectious causes
- Pyrexia is considered a protective mechanism in some situations, e.g. infection
- It can be life-threatening, e.g. malignant hyperthermia

Medical Student Survival Skills: The Acutely Ill Patient, First Edition. Philip Jevon, Konnur Ramkumar, and Emma Jenkinson.
© 2020 John Wiley & Sons Ltd. Published 2020 by John Wiley & Sons Ltd.
Companion website: www.wiley.com/go/jevon/medicalstudent

NB Pyrexia is a common clinical finding in acute illness.

 NB Normal body temperature ranges from about 36 to 37.5 °C.

Normal fluctuations in body temperature

- Circadian cycles (biological processes occurring naturally over a 24 hour period); the lowest temperature being recorded between 1 a.m. and 7 a.m. and highest between 4 p.m. and 11 p.m.
- Age, particularly in babies (ineffective thermoregulation)
- Exertion/exercise
- Menstrual cycle
- Ingestion of food
- Ambient temperature

Causes

- Infection (50% of cases): pyrogens (fever-producing proteins) are released by monocytes and macrophages (phagocytic cells responsible for the body's defence system); they act upon the thermoregulation centre in the hypothalamus, resulting in a rise in body temperature (due to an increase in heat production and a reduction in heat loss)
- High ambient temperature
- Drugs: e.g. amphetamine derivatives such as methylene dioxymetham-phetamine (ecstasy) or prescribed drugs such as some antidepressants/antipsychotics
- Allergy: e.g. reaction to a blood transfusion
- Stroke: injury to the hypothalamus
- Increased muscular activity: e.g. following strenuous exercise (particularly in a hot environment) and epilepsy
- Endocrine: e.g. thyroid storm (increased thyroid activity)
- Myocardial infarction

Pyrexia of unknown origin

- Pyrexia of unknown origin can be defined as a consistently elevated body temperature >37.5 °C persisting for longer than 2 weeks with no diagnosis despite initial investigations

- Causes include infection (30%), malignancy (20%), connective tissue disorders (e.g. Still's disease) (15%), and miscellaneous (e.g. inflammatory bowel disease) (20%); in 15% of cases either no diagnosis is made or the pyrexia resolves spontaneously

> ### OSCE Key Learning Points
>
> ✔ The most common cause of pyrexia is infection

Adverse effects associated with pyrexia

- Increased metabolic rate, oxygen consumption (10% increase with each 1 °C rise in temperature) and production of carbon dioxide
- Hypovolaemia due to sweating, dehydration, and vasodilation
- Metabolic acidosis
- Epilepsy
- Neurological impairment
- Renal failure
- Rhabdomyolysis
- Death

Treatment of pyrexia

- ABCDE
- If necessary summon expert help, administer high concentration oxygen, and treat life-threatening problems
- If necessary, obtain blood cultures and specimens for culture, e.g. urine and sputum
- Life-threatening hyperpyrexia: administer physical cooling methods
- Do not routinely administer antipyretic drugs, e.g. aspirin
- If able, try to establish the probable cause of the pyrexia (see investigations below)
- Make the patient comfortable, e.g. use of a fan, opening a window, and removing bed linen may be helpful

Investigations: The 6 'C's

- **C**hest: chest infection, patient coughing, breathless, productive cough, or purulent sputum? If necessary, obtain a sputum sample for microbiology, culture, and sensitivity

- **C**annula: site infected? (erythematous and painful)
- **C**alves: deep vein thrombosis? (tenderness, warmth, and hardness)
- **C**atheter/urine: urinary tract infection, urine foul smelling, cloudy? Has the patient got dysuria? Frequency?
- **C**ut: infected wound?
- **C**entral venous catheter: is the central venous catheter site infected?

Relevant blood tests for inflammatory markers

- White blood cell (WBC) count: a rise in the WBC count can indicate infection. The normal WBC range is 4.0–11.0
- C-reactive protein (CRP): an increase in CRP is significant. The normal CRP is $<6\,mg\,l^{-1}$
- Erythrocyte sedimentation rate (ESR): this is a test that measures the rate at which red blood cells settle out of suspension in blood plasma. In infection, the rate is quicker because the amount of protein in the blood increases. The normal ESR is 2–12 mm in 1 hour (Westergren's method) (this varies with age and is higher in women than men)

NB Routine use of physical cooling methods, e.g. tepid sponging and fanning, to reduce temperature has historically been very controversial. If the body's natural defence mechanism to combat infection is to increase body temperature, why try and reduce body temperature?

NB Antipyretics, e.g. aspirin or paracetamol, are not routinely recommended because they are unlikely to be effective and can mask the symptoms of illness.

Management of pyrexia in special circumstances

- *Pyrexia and the neutropenic patient*: the patient is usually actively treated with antibiotic therapy
- *Malignant hyperthermia*: a rare but potentially fatal complication of anaesthesia; characterised by a rapid rise in temperature, increased muscle

rigidity, tachycardia, and acidosis. The treatment is dantrolene administered by rapid IV injection

- *Sudden pyrexia associated with an IV infusion* (including transfusion of a blood product): this could indicate an allergic reaction. Stop the infusion, assess the patient following the ABCDE approach, and seek expert help/advice
- *Pyrexia in infants and children*: pyrexia is aa common symptom encountered in infants, children, and young persons, often indicating a self-limiting viral infection, rather than a bacterial or serious illness

8 Management of anaphylaxis

Definition: Severe, life-threatening, generalised, or systemic hypersensitivity reaction characterised by a compromised airway, breathing, and/or circulatory compromise; skin changes are usually present.

Incidence

- Since 1990, admissions for anaphylaxis have increased by 700%
- More common in females (60%) than in males (40%)
- Mean age for suffering anaphylaxis is 37 years
- 1 : 1333 of the English population have had anaphylaxis
- Risk of recurrent anaphylaxis reactions is 1 : 12

Deaths associated with anaphylaxis

- There are 20 anaphylaxis-related deaths each year in the UK
- Mortality rates are higher in patients with pre-existing asthma (particularly if poorly controlled)
- Fatal anaphylaxis: death usually occurs very soon after exposure to the trigger (Box 8.1)
- There are no reported deaths in anaphylaxis occurring >6 hours following exposure to trigger

Box 8.1 Association between exposure to common triggers and fatal anaphylaxis

- IV medication: typically 5 minutes later
- Insect stings: typically 10–15 minutes later (circulatory shock)
- Foodstuff: typically 30–35 minutes later (respiratory arrest)

Medical Student Survival Skills: The Acutely Ill Patient, First Edition. Philip Jevon, Konnur Ramkumar, and Emma Jenkinson.
© 2020 John Wiley & Sons Ltd. Published 2020 by John Wiley & Sons Ltd.
Companion website: www.wiley.com/go/jevon/medicalstudent

Pathophysiology

Mast cells and basophils release histamines and other vasoactive mediators that produce circulatory, respiratory, gastrointestinal, and cutaneous effects, e.g. pharyngeal and laryngeal oedema, bronchospasm, decreased vascular tone and capillary leak causing circulatory collapse.

Causes

Causes include:
- Drugs, e.g. penicillin, aspirin, anaesthetics
- Food products, e.g. peanuts, tree nuts (e.g. almonds, walnuts, cashews, Brazil nuts), sesame seeds, fish, shellfish, dairy products, eggs
- Bee/wasp stings
- Blood products
- 40% of anaphylactic reactions are idiopathic

Signs and symptoms

Signs and symptoms may include:
- Anxiety and feeling of impending doom
- Urticaria (Figure 8.1) and/or angioedema (Figure 8.2); skin changes are often the first sign, and are present in >80% of cases (Box 8.2)
- Respiratory distress: tachypnoea, wheeze, stridor
- Cardiovascular shock: tachycardia, hypotension, pallor
- Gastrointestinal symptoms, e.g. abdominal cramps, vomiting, and diarrhoea

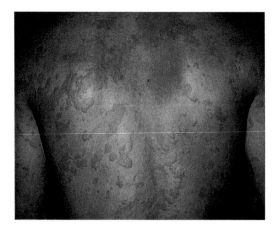

Figure 8.1 Urticaria.

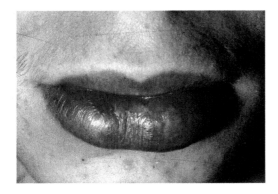

Figure 8.2 Angioedema.

Box 8.2 Skin/mucosal changes usually seen in anaphylaxis

- *Erythema*: patchy or generalised red rash
- *Urticaria* (hives, nettle rash, weals, or welts): different shapes and sizes, usually surrounded by a red flare and often itchy
- *Angioedema* (swelling of deeper tissues): usually in eyelids and lips; sometimes in mouth and throat

Diagnosis

The diagnosis of anaphylaxis is more likely if three criteria are met:
- Sudden onset; quick progression of symptoms
- Life-threatening A, B, and/or C problems
- Skin and/or mucosal changes

NB Skin and/or mucosal changes alone are not a sign of anaphylaxis. Likewise, patients may present with circulatory collapse/GI upset, without any airway or breathing compromise.

 Common misinterpretations and pitfalls

It is possible to mistake a panic or vasovagal attack for anaphylaxis. Remember the following differences:
- *Panic attack*: hyperventilation, tachycardia, and anxiety-related erythematous rash, but no hypotension, pallor, wheeze, or urticarial rash
- *Vasovagal attack*: the absence of a rash, tachycardia, and dyspnoea should rule out anaphylaxis as the cause of the collapse

ABCDE

Important signs and symptoms:

- *Airway*: hoarse voice, feeling of throat closing up, respiratory distress, difficulty in swallowing; stridor is a severe adverse sign
- *Breathing*: respiratory distress, tachypnoea, wheeze, confusion (due to hypoxia), tiredness; cyanosis is a late sign
- *Circulation*: tachycardia, hypotension, syncope, pallor, clammy skin, prolonged capillary refill time
- *Disability*: altered level of consciousness, e.g. confusion due to hypoxia
- *Exposure*: skin and/or mucosal changes (Box 8.2)

Emergency treatment of anaphylaxis

Emergency treatment of anaphylaxis should follow the Resuscitation Council (UK) anaphylaxis algorithm (Figure 8.3). Treatment can be divided up into first line and second line.

First line treatment

- Reassure the patient and call for help from senior colleagues (ring 2222?); a senior anaesthetist is required if the patient has stridor
- If possible, stop or remove the probable cause of the anaphylaxis
- Assess and treat the patient following the ABCDE approach
- Assist the patient into a comfortable position: flat with legs raised if in shock; upright if in respiratory distress
- Administer high-flow oxygen 15 l min⁻¹ via a non-rebreathe mask with an oxygen reservoir bag
- Administer adrenaline 500 µg (0.5 ml of 1 : 1000 solution) IM into the antero-lateral aspect of the middle third of the thigh (use a green [21G] or blue [23G] needle) (Box 8.3). This may be repeated at 5 minute intervals if there is no improvement in the patient's condition

NB Two strengths of adrenaline are available: 1 : 1000 solution (1 ml) and 1 : 10 000 (10 ml). The 1 : 1000 solution is used for IM injection in anaphylaxis.

- Ensure the patient has a clear airway; if stridor develops, alert senior expert help immediately (in anaphylaxis, stridor probably indicates the development of potentially life-threatening laryngeal oedema)

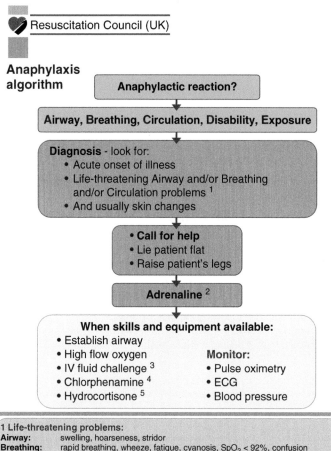

Resuscitation Council (UK)

Anaphylaxis algorithm

Anaphylactic reaction?

↓

Airway, Breathing, Circulation, Disability, Exposure

↓

Diagnosis - look for:
- Acute onset of illness
- Life-threatening Airway and/or Breathing and/or Circulation problems [1]
- And usually skin changes

↓

- **Call for help**
- Lie patient flat
- Raise patient's legs

↓

Adrenaline [2]

↓

When skills and equipment available:
- Establish airway
- High flow oxygen
- IV fluid challenge [3]
- Chlorphenamine [4]
- Hydrocortisone [5]

Monitor:
- Pulse oximetry
- ECG
- Blood pressure

---

1 Life-threatening problems:

Airway:	swelling, hoarseness, stridor
Breathing:	rapid breathing, wheeze, fatigue, cyanosis, SpO_2 < 92%, confusion
Circulation:	pale, clammy, low blood pressure, faintness, drowsy/coma

---

2 Adrenaline *(give IM unless experienced with IV adrenaline)*
IM doses of 1:1000 adrenaline (repeat after 5 min if no better)
- Adult   500 micrograms IM (0.5 mL)
- Child more than 12 years: 500 micrograms IM (0.5 mL)
- Child 6–12 years: 300 micrograms IM (0.3 mL)
- Child less than 6 years: 150 micrograms IM (0.15 mL)

Adrenaline IV to be given **only by experienced specialists**
Titrate: Adults 50 micrograms; Children 1 microgram/kg

3 IV fluid challenge:

Adult - 500–1000 mL
Child - crystalloid 20 mL/kg

Stop IV colloid
if this might be the cause
of anaphylaxis

---

	4 Chlorphenamine (IM or slow IV)	5 Hydrocortisone (IM or slow IV)
Adult or child more than 12 years	10 mg	200 mg
Child 6–12 years	5 mg	100 mg
Child 6 months to 6 years	2.5 mg	50 mg
Child less than 6 months	250 micrograms/kg	25 mg

Figure 8.3 Resuscitation Council (UK) anaphylaxis algorithm.

- Establish monitoring, e.g. pulse oximetry, electrocardiogram (ECG), blood pressure

 NB IV adrenaline in anaphylaxis is hazardous and should be administered by specialist practitioners only.

Second line treatment
- Insert a wide bore IV cannula (e.g. 14 G)
- Administer fluid challenge: 500–1000 ml (e.g. 0.9% normal saline) and monitor response
- Administer chlorpheniramine 10 mg IM or slow IV (may prevent histamine-mediated vasodilation and bronchoconstriction)
- Administer hydrocortisone 200 mg IM or slow IV (may prevent or shorten protracted reactions)
- Consider bronchodilator therapy, e.g. salbutamol (inhaled or IV), ipratropium (inhaled), aminophylline (IV), or magnesium (IV)
- Assess and reassess following ABCDE approach
- Do not sit or stand patient up as this could cause deterioration
- Reassure patient

Box 8.3 Benefits of adrenaline

- Reverses peripheral vasodilation
- Reduces oedema
- Dilates the airways
- Increases myocardial contractility
- Suppresses histamine and leukotriene release.

Investigations

- Routine bloods
- Peak expiratory flow measurement
- Arterial blood gas analysis
- 12 lead ECG
- Chest X-ray
- Mast cell tryptase: ideally take three samples – as soon as possible, after 1–2 hours, and 24 hours or later (patient's baseline)

Cardiopulmonary arrest

- Perform standard advanced life support (ALS) procedures including early tracheal intubation
- Administer adrenaline IV (not IM)
- Consider steroids, antihistamines (if not already administered), and large volumes of IV fluids

 Uncommon presentations

Anaphylaxis can present without skin changes.

OSCE Key Learning Points

Initial treatment of anaphylaxis

✔ Diagnosis: acute onset, skin changes, compromised A, B, and/or C

✔ Call for senior help early (SBAR)

✔ Position patient appropriately

✔ Administer oxygen 15 l min^{-1}

✔ Administer adrenaline 500 µg (0.5 ml of 1 : 1000 solution) IM

Management of acute asthma

Z Kimbley

Manor Hospital, Walsall, UK

> **Definition:** Asthma is an inflammatory condition causing reversible airway obstruction with symptoms of cough, wheeze, and shortness of breath.

Background

- Acute exacerbations are associated with an increase in symptoms and deterioration in peak flow
- Exacerbations can be classified as moderate, severe, life-threatening, or near fatal (see Box 9.1)
- 5.1 million people in the UK receive treatment for asthma
- 8% have had an emergency admission for asthma in the last year

Asthma deaths

- 1400 people die from asthma each year in the UK
- The majority of people who die from asthma have chronically severe asthma rather than a severe attack in those with mild or moderate disease
- Most deaths occur before admission to hospital
- The best strategy is early recognition and intervention

Pathophysiology

Reversible airway obstruction is caused by:
- Bronchial muscle contraction

Medical Student Survival Skills: The Acutely Ill Patient, First Edition. Philip Jevon, Konnur Ramkumar, and Emma Jenkinson.
© 2020 John Wiley & Sons Ltd. Published 2020 by John Wiley & Sons Ltd.
Companion website: www.wiley.com/go/jevon/medicalstudent

- Mucosal inflammation: mast cell and basophil degranulation leads to inflammatory mediator release
- Increased mucus production

Causes and triggers

- Exercise
- Allergen exposure – pollen, dust mite, pets
- Occupational – dust, dye, resin
- Medications, e.g. beta-blockers, non-steroidal anti-inflammatory drugs (NSAIDs), aspirin, adenosine

Symptoms

- Wheeze
- Shortness of breath (SOB)
- Chest tightness
- Cough

Signs

- Look for signs of respiratory distress: use of accessory muscles, difficulty completing sentences
- Count respiratory rate: is there tachypnoea?
- Check trachea position: is it central?
- Check chest expansion: is it equal?
- Check pulse: is there tachycardia?
- Auscultate the chest for wheeze and check for bilateral air entry (*think pneumothorax*); a silent chest becomes more common as the attack becomes more severe

Diagnosis

- An acute exacerbation of asthma is diagnosed by the presence of worsening symptoms and/or deterioration in peak expiratory flow (PEF)
- An attack can be graded on severity (Box 9.1)

Box 9.1 Severity grading of asthma

Moderate
- Increasing symptoms
- PEF >50–75% best or predicted
- No features of acute severe asthma

Acute severe
- PEF 33–50% best or predicted
- Respiratory rate $\geq 25\,min^{-1}$
- Heart rate $\geq 110\,bpm$
- Inability to complete sentences in one breath

Life-threatening
- PEF <33% best or predicted
- SpO_2 <92%
- PaO_2 <8 kPa
- Normal $PaCO_2$ (4.6–6.0 kPa)
- Silent chest
- Cyanosis
- Poor respiratory effort
- Arrhythmia
- Exhaustion, altered conscious level

Near fatal
- Raised $PaCO_2$ and/or requiring mechanical ventilation with raised inflation pressures

Differential diagnosis

- Exacerbation of chronic obstructive pulmonary disease
- Pulmonary embolism
- Pulmonary oedema
- Anaphylaxis

ABCDE

- *Airway*: can the patient talk, is their airway patent
- *Breathing*: tachypnoea, wheeze, respiratory distress. Cyanosis, exhaustion, and silent chest are late signs
- *Circulation*: tachycardia initially, bradycardia is a late sign
- *Disability*: confusion or altered level of consciousness due to hypoxia
- *Exposure*: temperature

Emergency treatment of acute asthma

Initial treatment

- ABCDE
- Sit upright
- Administer oxygen: initially high flow 15 l min^{-1}, and once stable target to maintain saturations at 94–98%
- Give nebulisers: bronchodilators, e.g. salbutamol 2.5–5 mg, may need to be given repeatedly every 15–30 minutes
- Secure IV access
- Give steroids: hydrocortisone 200 mg IV or prednisolone 40 mg orally
- Discuss with senior or intensive treatment unit (ITU) early if there are life-threatening features
- Review after 15–30 minutes of treatment (Box 9.2)

Patient improving

- Continue oxygen therapy and target saturations at 94–98%
- Prednisolone 40 mg once daily
- Nebulised salbutamol 5 mg 4–6 hourly
- Repeat peak flow 6 hourly

Patient not improving

- Continue oxygen and nebulisers as above
- Add nebulised ipratropium bromide 500 µg 4–6 hourly
- Consider magnesium sulphate (1.2–2 g IV over 20 minutes) (after consultation with senior medical staff)
- Involve seniors and ITU
- Can consider IV aminophylline/IV salbutamol

Box 9.2 Treatment review

- Reassess patient 15–30 minutes after treatment
- Use ABCDE approach
- Focus on:
  - Oxygen saturation
  - PEF
  - Arterial blood gas

Indications for admission to ITU

- Patients requiring ventilation
- Those with severe or life-threatening asthma with failing medical therapy:
  - Worsening hypoxia
  - Deteriorating peak flow
  - Hypercapnia
  - Acidosis on arterial blood gases
  - Exhaustion: feeble respiration, silent chest
  - Altered conscious level
  - Respiratory arrest

 Common misinterpretations and pitfalls

Antibiotics should only be given if there is evidence of bacterial infection; most exacerbations of asthma are likely to be viral and the role of bacterial infection is often overestimated.

Investigations

- Oxygen saturations
- Routine bloods
- 12 lead electrocardiogram (ECG)
- Arterial blood gases
- Peak flow:
  - ≤33% of best or predicted – life-threatening exacerbation
  - ≤50% of best or predicted – severe exacerbation
  - 50–75% of best or predicted – moderate exacerbation

Cardiopulmonary arrest

- Cardiac arrest in asthma is usually a terminal event after a period of hypoxia
- The factors involved are:
  - Cardiac arrhythmias due to hypoxia, electrolyte abnormalities, and stimulant drugs, e.g. beta-agonists
  - Bronchospasm and mucous plugging leading to asphyxia
  - Tension pneumothorax

NB A chest X-ray is not indicated for all acute asthma patients, but consider it if there is:
- Suspected pneumothorax
- Suspected consolidation
- Life-threatening asthma
- Failure to respond to initial treatment
- Need for ventilation

- In case of cardiac arrest follow basic life support (BLS) and advanced life support (ALS) protocols
- Use early intubation
- Look for reversible causes

 Uncommon presentations

Remember that there is an increased risk of pneumothorax in asthmatics, and consider tension pneumothorax if very unwell. Pneumothorax can be bilateral.

Discharge checklist

- Follow up within 2 working days by a GP
- Check the patient's inhaler technique before discharge
- Give the patient a peak flow meter to use at home
- Give the patient a written asthma management plan

NB The British Thoracic Society recommend that following an episode of acute asthma patients should be treated for at least 5 days, or until recovery. Short courses of oral corticosteroids of up to 2 weeks can be stopped abruptly.

OSCE Key Learning Points

✔ Diagnosis: deterioration in PEF, SOB, and wheeze
✔ Administer oxygen
✔ Administer salbutamol nebulisers and steroids
✔ Be aware that deterioration can be rapid, so get early senior and ITU input

10 Management of hypovolaemia

> **Definition:** Hypovolaemia refers to a state of reduced blood volume.

Background

- This is the commonest cause of shock (see Box 10.1 for other causes)

Box 10.1 Causes of shock

- *Hypovolaemic shock*
- *Distributive shock* – results from an increased volume of distribution ('relative hypovolaemia'), e.g. toxin release and vasodilation in sepsis or anaphylaxis, or loss of sympathetic vasomotor control in spinal injury
- *Cardiogenic shock* – due to primary pump (cardiac) failure
- *Obstructive shock* – due to obstruction of cardiac output (e.g. tension pneumothorax, massive pulmonary embolus, or cardiac tamponade)

- Hypovolaemia can be defined using parameters such as systolic blood pressure (BP) or central venous pressure
- Alternatively, it can be identified by signs of decreased organ perfusion, e.g. delayed capillary refill, confusion, or reduced urine output
- Hypovolaemia differs slightly from *dehydration*, which involves fluid loss and consequent hypernatraemia; hypovolaemia usually involves sodium *and* water loss
- Shock is usually categorised into four classes (Box 10.2)

Medical Student Survival Skills: The Acutely Ill Patient, First Edition. Philip Jevon, Konnur Ramkumar, and Emma Jenkinson.
© 2020 John Wiley & Sons Ltd. Published 2020 by John Wiley & Sons Ltd.
Companion website: www.wiley.com/go/jevon/medicalstudent

> ## Box 10.2 Classes of shock
>
> - *Class I* – up to 15% volume loss: usually no clinical signs or symptoms
> - *Class II* – up to 30% volume loss: postural drop in BP, decreased pulse pressure, slight tachycardia, subtle increase in respiratory rate, mildly anxious
> - *Class III* – up to 40% volume loss: tachycardia, tachypnoea, slightly decreased systolic BP, decreased urine output, anxious and confused
> - *Class IV* – more than 40% volume loss: tachycardia, tachypnoea, decreased systolic BP, markedly decreased urine output, confused/lethargic

> ## OSCE Key Learning Points
>
> ✔ The classification of shock follows the scoring in tennis: 0%, 15%, 30%, and 40%

Causes

- Blood loss (haemorrhagic shock) (Box 10.3)
- Plasma loss (e.g. in burns)

> ## Box 10.3 Sources of haemorrhage
>
> - *Overt* – external wounds, bleeding varicose vein, haematemesis or melaena, rectal or vaginal bleeding
> - *Occult* – closed injuries in trauma (chest, abdomen, pelvis or long bones), gastrointestinal blood loss, ruptured aortic aneurysm, retroperitoneal haematoma
> - Remember to consider coagulopathies (including iatrogenic, e.g. warfarin)

Pathophysiology

- A decreased blood volume initially causes a compensatory response: the heart rate increases to improve cardiac output, and peripheral vasoconstriction occurs to preserve peripheral vascular resistance and to maintain perfusion to essential organs

- No decrease in BP occurs until relatively late because of these compensatory mechanisms

 Common misinterpretations and pitfalls

Signs of hypovolaemia may be masked in those who are very physically fit (e.g. professional athletes), those with pacemakers, or in patients who take medications such as beta-blockers.

ABCDE

Important signs and symptoms include:
- *Airway*
- *Breathing*: tachypnea is usually present
- *Circulation*: tachycardia, reduction/loss of pulse volume, hypotension, pallor, clammy skin, prolonged capillary refill time, oliguria
- *Disability*: altered level of consciousness, e.g. confusion and drowsiness due to poor cerebral perfusion
- *Exposure*: pale clammy skin; evidence of blood loss, e.g. drain

Emergency treatment of hypovolaemia

- Assess and treat the patient following the ABCDE approach
- Assist the patient into a comfortable position: normally lying flat with the legs raised
- Administer high-flow oxygen 15 l min^{-1} via a non-rebreathe mask with an oxygen reservoir bag
- Establish monitoring, e.g. pulse oximetry, electrocardiogram (ECG), BP; central venous pressure monitoring and bedside ultrasound assessment of inferior vena cava diameter are also effective and relatively straightforward but do require specialist input
- Secure IV access. Patients with hypovolaemia should have good IV access as soon as possible: ideally, this would be two wide bore cannulas in large veins. However, in patients who are significantly shut down, early intraosseous access should be considered
- Administer fluid challenge: 500–1000 ml (e.g. 0.9% normal saline) and monitor response
- Assess and reassess following ABCDE approach

Common misinterpretations and pitfalls

- Non-invasive BP readings are only valid at the time when they were taken and need to be measured regularly, even on 'continuous monitoring', whereas pulse rate and oxygen saturation levels are measured beat-to-beat
- Most machines allow you to select the frequency with which non-invasive BP readings are checked, so for unwell patients ensure that BP measurements are recorded on a regular basis, e.g. every 5 or 15 minutes

- Monitor urine output (preferably via a urinary catheter and an hourly measurement bag); this is a useful parameter and does not require any specialist input
- Order appropriate investigations, e.g. ECG and chest X-ray. Any suggestion of underlying heart disease, pulmonary oedema, or acute respiratory distress syndrome (ARDS) should prompt caution with fluids and early senior/specialist input. A venous gas sample will provide several useful parameters quickly (Box 10.4) and any patient with evidence of significant blood loss should have a blood or marrow sample sent for cross matching as soon as possible, plus baseline full blood count, renal function, and clotting samples

Box 10.4 Information available from venous blood gas samples

Most machines will give you the following parameters useful in the assessment of shock:

- Electrolytes (may be altered by medication, dehydration, etc.)
- Haemoglobin (may be lowered in haemorrhagic shock)
- Lactate (may be elevated in any state of significant shock)
- pH (may be lowered in a shocked/dehydrated patient)
  Glucose (may be reduced *or* elevated in significant shock)

 Common misinterpretations and pitfalls

It is easy to be falsely reassured by a normal BP; however remember that hypotension is a late sign of shock, not seen in classes I or II. Pay close heed to the pulse and respiratory rates, pulse pressure, and the mental state of the patient. Patients who are young and physically fit are able to compensate for hypovolaemia and may maintain normal physiological parameters until they are severely hypovolaemic.

Treatment of hypovolaemia

There are essentially three management options: replace the volume, tighten the system, or reverse the cause.

- *Replace the volume*: can use crystalloid-type fluids, colloid-type fluids, or blood/blood products (Box 10.5). A fluid challenge of appropriate volume should be given and the response assessed: the volume will depend on the size, age, and co-morbidities of a patient. It is usually appropriate to give an initial fluid challenge of 500 ml

---

Box 10.5 Fluid products

Numerous fluid replacement products are available, and usually broadly divided into crystalloids or colloids.

- *Crystalloids* (e.g. 0.9% saline or Hartmann's solution) are the most appropriate first line fluid for resuscitation; there is no role for 5% dextrose as a resuscitation fluid as this is redistributed too rapidly
- *Colloids* (e.g. Gelofusin, Volulyte, Voluplex) are frequently used as second line fluids for resuscitation, although there is no clear evidence that they are superior to crystalloids – senior support should be sought
- Blood products should be considered early, particularly in those with haemorrhage, or those receiving large volumes of fluid, e.g. in septic shock

---

- *Tighten the system*: vasoconstriction can be achieved using inotropic agents; this requires senior/specialist input
- *Reverse the cause*: ultimately the best treatment option is to reverse the cause; this requires early identification, plus consultation with the appropriate specialist

 NB Identify and correct coagulopathies in patients who have received significant fluid resuscitation.

Management of sepsis

B Taylor

Manor Hospital, Walsall, UK

Definition: The definition of sepsis is a progressive hierarchy, from sepsis, through severe sepsis to septic shock. Systemic inflammatory response syndrome (SIRS) is a collection of symptoms which have a number of causes, only one of which is sepsis (Box 11.1).

Box 11.1 Sepsis and SIRS

- *SIRS*: a systemic inflammatory condition characterised by two or more of:
  - Temperature greater than 38 C or less than 36 C
  - Heart rate greater than 90 bpm
  - Respiratory rate greater than 20, or $PaCO_2$ less than 4.3 kPa
  - White cell count less than 4 or greater than 12×10^9 l^{-1}
- *Sepsis*: SIRS with suspected or proven infection
- *Severe sepsis*: sepsis with organ dysfunction or tissue hypoperfusion (hypotension, raised lactate, or decreased urine output)
- *Septic shock*: severe sepsis with persistently low blood pressure despite intravenous fluid resuscitation

Incidence

- Sepsis is an extremely common presentation to multiple hospital specialties
- Septic shock is the second most common cause of death in intensive treatment units (ITUs)
- Sepsis accounts for 25% of ITU admissions
- It is more common and severe in patients with immunosuppression

Medical Student Survival Skills: The Acutely Ill Patient, First Edition. Philip Jevon, Konnur Ramkumar, and Emma Jenkinson.
© 2020 John Wiley & Sons Ltd. Published 2020 by John Wiley & Sons Ltd.
Companion website: www.wiley.com/go/jevon/medicalstudent

Prognosis

- There is 20–35% mortality from severe sepsis
- There is 30–70% mortality from septic shock
- On the other hand, mild sepsis is extremely common, and is usually treated in the community with oral antibiotics and would be expected to resolve completely
- Therefore, clinical alertness and suspicion should be kept in case of deterioration, and 'safety netting' should always be used (encourage the patient or their carer to return if they have any concerns)
- Have a low threshold for referral and treatment where risk factors exist (Box 11.2)

Box 11.2 Risk factors for severe sepsis/septic shock

- *Extremes of age*: the very young and very old are at high risk
- *Immunocompromise*: neutropenia, chemotherapy, immunosuppressants, steroids, splenectomy, acquired immune deficiency syndrome (AIDS)
- *Concurrent critical illness or injury*: burns, critical care admission, major trauma
- *Indwelling devices*: cannulas, lines, and anything that bypasses surface defences

---

Pathophysiology

- SIRS: uncontrolled release of inflammatory cytokines leading to cytokine storm, triggered by infection (sepsis) or tissue injury (e.g. burns, surgery)
- Gram-negative bacteria (e.g. *Neisseria meningitidis*) release endotoxins when lysed, which can trigger a massive SIRS response
- Gram-positive bacteria (e.g. *Staphylococcus aureus*) can produce exotoxins, e.g. toxic shock syndrome

Signs and symptoms

Signs and symptoms can be divided into general signs of systemic sepsis and local signs of a specific infection:

General signs
- Acute or subacute onset
- Hypotension

- Tachycardia
- Tachypnoea
- Mottled skin
- Non-blanching purpuric rash
- Cool peripheries (occasionally warm, dilated peripheries in early stages)
- Pyrexia (in severe sepsis/shock, often hypothermia)
- Confusion

Specific signs of infection

- Meningitis – Kernig's sign, neck rigidity, photophobia
- Pneumonia – productive cough, focal chest signs, pleuritic chest pain
- Endocarditis – new murmur, embolic phenomena (e.g. splinter haemorrhages, microscopic haematuria)
- Intra-abdominal sepsis – guarding, abdominal signs
- Urosepsis – tender renal angles, dysuria, pyuria
- Cellulitis – rash. A rapidly spreading rash is necrotising fasciitis until proven otherwise!

Investigations

 NB If severe sepsis is suspected *do not* delay antibiotic treatment to fully investigate.

- Serum lactate (many blood gas machines will measure lactate)
- Arterial or venous blood gas
- Blood cultures if possible. *If these are not easy to take, do not delay antibiotic administration*
- White cell count
- C-reactive protein (beware of a lag effect). This is less useful as a single measurement, but the trend can be useful to monitor response to treatment
- Identification of source:
  - Chest X-ray
  - Urinalysis followed by urine microscopy, culture and sensitivity (MC&S) if indicated. Follow local guidance on catheter specimens as these may often throw up contaminants of no clinical significance
  - Sputum cultures
  - If meningitis is suspected – computed tomography (CT) of head, lumbar puncture

- If endocarditis is suspected – echocardiography (initially transthoracic, but a transoesophageal echo may be required)
- If intra-abdominal sepsis is suspected – CT or ultrasound of abdomen
- Seek specialist advice if there is an indwelling foreign object (e.g. shunts, synthetic grafts, prosthetic joints or valves)

 Common misinterpretations and pitfalls

- *Not all SIRS is sepsis.* Pancreatitis often presents in a similar way to sepsis, and has similar clinical and biochemical changes
- *Sepsis can present with a low temperature.* These are often the sickest septic patients and a delay in their diagnosis because fever is absent can be fatal
- *Some forms of sepsis need emergency surgery.* Necrotising fasciitis and severe intra-abdominal sepsis require surgical control of the source and warrant immediate surgical referral
- *Not every positive culture implies infection.* Cultures are commonly 'contaminated' with normal skin flora. This will result in a false-positive culture. Meticulous aseptic technique is therefore important when taking blood cultures. However, repeated cultures showing the same 'contaminant' bacteria may actually be due to endocarditis

ABCDE assessment

Important signs and symptoms include:
- *Airway*: loss of airway is usually secondary to loss of consciousness due to shock or meningitis. Epiglottitis is a specific form of sepsis affecting the airway
- *Breathing*: tachypnoea is an early sign. Oxygen saturations may not read if there is poor peripheral perfusion. Severe pneumonia may result in profound hypoxaemia
- *Circulation*: there may be hypotension with tachycardia. Peripheries may be warm initially (vasodilation), but in severe sepsis they become cool and shut down. Capillary refill may be delayed
- *Disability*: there may be agitation and confusion (particularly in elderly) due to pyrexia and shock. Loss of consciousness either suggests meningitis or profound shock. Blood glucose may rise due to the stress response and may fall in later stages
- *Exposure*: look carefully for rashes or signs of necrotising fasciitis. Examine the abdomen

Emergency treatment of sepsis

 NB The 'sepsis six' (Box 11.3).

Box 11.3 The sepsis six

1 Administer high-flow oxygen (if oxygen saturations are <94%)
2 Take blood cultures
3 Administer empirical IV antibiotics
4 Measure serum lactate and send full blood count
5 Start IV fluid resuscitation
6 Commence accurate urine output measurement

- Assess and treat the patient following the ABCDE approach
- Call for help early: SBAR
- Assist the patient into a comfortable position: normally lying flat with the legs raised
- Administer high-flow oxygen 15 l min^{-1} via a non-rebreathe mask with an oxygen reservoir bag
- Establish monitoring, e.g. pulse oximetry, electrocardiogram (ECG), blood pressure; central venous pressure monitoring and bedside ultrasound assessment of inferior vena cava diameter are also effective and relatively straightforward but do require specialist input
- Take blood cultures as soon as possible. Other important tests include chest X-ray, ECG, lactate, full blood count, and urea and electrolytes (U&Es)
- Secure IV access: ideally, this would be two wide bore cannulas in the large veins
- Commence fluid resuscitation. Administer boluses of 500–1000 ml and monitor response
- Insert urinary catheter and closely monitor urine output
- Administer antibiotics early (within an hour), according to local antimicrobial guidelines.
- Monitor blood gases: venous gases are usually adequate unless the patient has respiratory distress or an oxygen requirement

NB Antibiotic administration is time critical.

- Consider early source control – 'if there's pus about, let it out!'. Request urine and sputum samples for MC&S
- Ensure early referral to critical care if severe sepsis or septic shock. Persistent hypotension despite fluid resuscitation is an indication for critical care

 Uncommon presentations

- Immunosuppressed patients may not demonstrate typical signs and symptoms until very late in the illness (as no inflammatory response is raised)
- Fungal infections may present late
- Viral infections can be severe and fulminant (e.g. pandemic influenza, severe acute respiratory syndrome/Middle East respiratory syndrome), or can be clinically similar to a similar bacterial infection (e.g. encephalitis)

OSCE Key Learning Points

✔ *Diagnosis*: acute/subacute onset; high or low temperature, tachycardia, hypotension, and tachypnoea; high or low white cell count
✔ *Treatment*: the 'sepsis six' (if required to maintain oxygen saturations >94%):
    1 High-flow oxygen
    2 Blood cultures
    3 Empirical IV antibiotics
    4 Serum lactate and full blood count
    5 IV fluid resuscitation
    6 Catheterise and monitor urine output

12 Management of acute stroke

Definition: Focal neurological deficit with a vascular cause:
- If it resolves <24 hours it is usually termed a transient ischaemic attack (TIA)
- If it lasts >24 hours it is classed as a stroke

OSCE Key Learning Points

✔ At the time of presentation it is not always possible to differentiate between a TIA and a stroke

Causes

- 80%: infarction (thrombosis, emboli, or hypoperfusion); the majority of which involve the middle cerebral artery
- 20%: haemorrhage

Signs and symptoms

- Signs and symptoms vary according to the area involved (Box 12.1)
- The 'FAST' test is a validated tool used to identify patients with probable stroke in the pre-hospital setting: '**F**ace, **A**rm, **S**peech, **T**ime to call 999
- Cerebellar and brainstem strokes can be difficult to diagnose and require a high index of suspicion. Patients may present with nausea, vomiting, vertigo, visual disturbance or ataxia

Medical Student Survival Skills: The Acutely Ill Patient, First Edition. Philip Jevon, Konnur Ramkumar, and Emma Jenkinson.
© 2020 John Wiley & Sons Ltd. Published 2020 by John Wiley & Sons Ltd.
Companion website: www.wiley.com/go/jevon/medicalstudent

Box 12.1 Overview of signs and symptoms in stroke (infarction)

- *Anterior cerebral artery*
  - Weakness/paralysis of contralateral leg > arm
  - Frontal lobe symptoms (e.g. disinhibition)
- *Middle cerebral artery (MCA)*
  - Symptoms depend on site: total MCA occlusion causes contralateral hemiplegia (arm > leg) and paraesthesia, plus ipsilateral homonymous hemianopia
  - Dominant hemisphere (usually left-sided) lesions cause dysphasia; non-dominant (right-sided) lesions often cause contralateral neglect
- *Posterior cerebral artery 'posterior circulation'*
  - Contralateral visual defects, amnesia, speech disturbance
- *Cerebellar*
  - Headache, nausea/vomiting, ataxia, dizziness/vertigo, nystagmus, dysarthria, reduced conscious level
- *Brainstem*
  - Headache, nausea/vomiting, vertigo, cranial nerve deficits, ataxia, weakness, nystagmus, dysarthria, altered conscious level, abnormal breathing patterns

 Common misinterpretations and pitfalls

Hypoglycaemia, hemiplegic migraine, and Todd's paresis are common presentations that can mimic a stroke.

Diagnosis

- Beware of 'stroke mimics' (Box 12.2)
- It is largely a clinical diagnosis based on the findings above
- Check bedside blood sugar to exclude hypoglycaemia
- Use the ROSIER (recognition of stroke in the emergency room) score (validated for use in hospitals) (Box 12.3)

Box 12.2 Stroke mimics

- *Common*
  - Hypoglycaemia
  - Hemiplegic migraine
  - Todd's paresis (focal neurology post seizure)
- *Less common*
  - Space-occupying lesions (tumours, abscesses)
  - Infections (encephalitis, abscesses)
  - Other intracranial haemorrhage (e.g. subdural haematoma)
  - Demyelinating disorders (e.g. multiple sclerosis)

Box 12.3 ROSIER score

- Has there been loss of consciousness/syncope? [Y] –1, [N] 0
- Has there been seizure activity? [Y] –1, [N] 0
- Is there a new onset (or on waking) of:
  - Asymmetrical facial weakness? [Y] +1, [N] 0
  - Asymmetrical arm weakness? [Y] +1, [N] 0
  - Asymmetrical leg weakness? [Y] +1, [N] 0
  - Speech disturbance? [Y] +1, [N] 0
  - Visual field defect? [Y] +1, [N] 0

Total score (–2 to +5)>0 means a stroke is likely, below this the possibility of stroke is lower but not excluded

Emergency treatment of acute stroke

- ABCDE
- Request monitoring, e.g. pulse oximetry, electrocardiogram (ECG), and non-invasive blood pressure (BP) monitoring
- Ensure patient has a clear airway; if patient has altered level of consciousness place in recovery (lateral position); if patient is unconscious, consider using an airway adjunct, e.g. oropharyngeal airway, and request expert help as advanced airway intervention, e.g. tracheal intubation, may be necessary

- Consider administering oxygen 15 l min^{-1} (guided by pulse oximetry)
- Closely monitor BP (hypertension may be present and indeed may be the underlying cause of the stroke); seek expert help if hypertension is present and BP control is required
- Record 12 lead ECG – look for atrial fibrillation (probable cause of blood clot causing ischaemic stroke)
- Check bedside blood glucose – hypoglycaemia can mimic the signs of a stroke
- Insert venous cannula and commence IV fluids
- Order appropriate investigations, e.g. bloods (including full blood count, urea and electrolytes (U&Es), glucose, international normalised ratio, and group and save), chest X-ray
- Keep nil by mouth pending swallowing assessment
- Order immediate computed tomography (CT) head scan where indicated, to exclude intracranial haemorrhage (Box 12.4)
- CT head scan within 24 hours in other patients
- Ensure the practitioner is trained in the use of the National Institutes of Health Stroke Scale (NIHSS) to assess the severity of symptoms
- Assess the need for cot sides

Box 12.4 Indications for immediate CT head (within 1 hour)

- Potentially suitable for thrombolysis
- Patient is anticoagulated or known to have a bleeding tendency
- Decreased Glasgow coma score (< 13)
- Progressive/fluctuating symptoms
- Papilloedema, neck stiffness, or fever
- Severe headache with onset of symptoms

Definitive treatment of stroke

- Contact stroke team as soon as possible
- Where indicated, thrombolysis (with alteplase) should be commenced as soon as possible (Box 12.5) – *usually by the stroke team*
- All patients (unless contraindicated) should have aspirin 300 mg daily (orally or rectally), with a proton pump inhibitor if gastro-protection is needed
- All patients should be admitted to a specialist stroke unit as soon as possible (within 4 hours of presentation)

Box 12.5 Thrombolysis with alteplase

Indications

- Clinical diagnosis of ischaemic stroke
- Patient aged <80 years and >18 years
- Treatment can be commenced within 4.5 hours of onset of symptoms
- Haemorrhagic stroke has been excluded

Contraindications

- Active internal bleeding
- Suspected aortic dissection
- Previous intracranial haemorrhage
- Ischaemic stroke or head injury in previous 3 months
- Seizure associated with stroke
- Current anticoagulated state
- Major surgery in previous 3 months
- Lumbar puncture in previous 7 days
- Pregnant during previous 1 month
- Central venous cannulation in previous 10 days
- Current vitreous bleed or retinopathy
- Major trauma or cardiopulmonary resuscitation in previous 1 month
- Recent myocardial infarction or current pericarditis
- Very mild or very severe stroke symptoms (NIHSS <4 or >25)
- Hypoglycaemia (<3) or uncontrolled hyperglycaemia (>22)
- Hypertension (systolic BP >185, diastolic BP >110)

Note that local protocols may vary

Treatment of TIA

- These patients are at high risk of further stroke and require careful risk stratification, using the ABCD^2 score (Box 12.6)
- Patients with high scores (see local guidelines) should be referred to the in-patient stroke team
- Those patients with low scores may be suitable for discharge but must be reviewed in a specialist clinic within 24 hours
- Patients should be commenced on 300 mg aspirin

- When discharging patients following a TIA do not forget to tell them (and document that you have done so) that they must not drive for 1 month: they do not need to inform the DVLA (UK Driver and Vehicle Licensing Agency)

Box 12.6 ABCD² score

Age: < 60 years = 0, ≥ 60 years = 1
Blood pressure: systolic BP ≤ 140 mmHg and/or diastolic BP ≤ 90 mmHg = 0, systolic BP > 140 mmHg and/or > 90 mmHg = 1
Clinical features: unilateral weakness = 2, speech disturbance without weakness = 1, other symptoms = 0
Duration of symptoms: < 10 minutes = 0, 10–59 minutes = 1, ≥ 60 minutes = 2
Diabetes: no = 0, yes = 1
Total score: 0–3 = low risk, 4–5 = moderate risk, 6–7 = high risk

OSCE Key Learning Points

✔ If patients present with loss of consciousness, confusion, seizures, or urinary incontinence, TIA is unlikely; consider an alternative diagnosis

Management of chest pain

Background

- Chest pain is one of the most common emergency presentations
- Nearly one in six men and one in 10 women die from coronary heart disease (CHD)
- Ischaemic heart disease (IHD) is the cause of 73 000 deaths in the UK each year (200 per day or one every 7 minutes)
- 2.3 million people are living with IHD in the UK (1.4 million men and 850 000 women)
- Death rates from CHD are higher in Scotland and the north of England and lower in the south of England

Signs and symptoms of acute coronary syndrome

Typical signs and symptoms of acute coronary syndrome (ACS) include:
- Central/retrosternal pain/heaviness/tightness
- Tight/crushing/heavy/burning pain
- Exertional pain, relieved by rest or nitrates
- Radiation of pain into neck, jaw, or left/both arm(s)
- Breathlessness
- Sweating
- Nausea or vomiting
- Pallor

Medical Student Survival Skills: The Acutely Ill Patient, First Edition. Philip Jevon, Konnur Ramkumar, and Emma Jenkinson.
© 2020 John Wiley & Sons Ltd. Published 2020 by John Wiley & Sons Ltd.
Companion website: www.wiley.com/go/jevon/medicalstudent

Chest pain: Differential diagnoses

- *Ischaemic heart disease* – acute coronary syndrome
- *Pulmonary embolism* – classically a sharp, pleuritic pain associated with breathlessness, in the presence or absence of symptoms of deep vein thrombosis or of risk factors for thromboembolic disease
- *Thoracic aortic dissection* – classically a tearing pain radiating through into the back
- *Pericarditis* – classically a sharp pain, worse on lying flat, associated with flu-like symptoms
- *Pneumothorax* – a sharp, pleuritic pain associated with breathlessness
- *Pneumonia* – usually pleuritic pain, associated with cough/fever
- *Oesophageal rupture* – severe retrosternal pain, often after forceful vomiting
- *Gastrointestinal* – e.g. reflux, pancreatitis, gallstones or peptic ulcer
- *Musculoskeletal* – usually sharp, pleuritic, worse on coughing/movement, and tender to touch
- *'Non-specific chest pain'* – this is a diagnosis of exclusion; chest pain of unknown cause may be precipitated by anxiety in some patients
- *Other* – shingles, metastatic rib disease, or radicular pain from spinal disease

Risk factors for IHD

Risk factors for IHD should be sought, including:
- Smoking
- Diabetes
- Hyperlipidaemia
- Increasing age
- Male sex
- Family history
- Life style (stress)
- Overweight
- Ethnicity

Spectrum of ACS presentations

- *Stable angina* – precipitated by exertion or cold weather, relieved by rest or glyceryl trinitrate (GTN) spray, and lasts 5–15 minutes

- *Unstable angina* – as above but symptoms persist or are triggered at rest; electrocardiogram (ECG) and cardiac enzymes are normal
- *Acute coronary syndrome* – as above; the ECG is normal and cardiac enzymes (typically high-sensitivity troponin) are elevated
- *Non-ST-elevation myocardial infarction (NSTEMI)* – as for ACS but new (or dynamic) ECG changes (e.g. T-wave inversion) are present
- *ST-elevation myocardial infarction (STEMI)* – ST segment elevation is present on the ECG

Diagnosis

- History
- 12 lead ECG
- Elevated troponin levels

NB Troponin levels are not diagnostic of ischaemic chest pain, rather they should be used for risk stratification and to guide urgency of management.

 Common misinterpretations and pitfalls

Posterior myocardial infarction is easily missed and should be considered in the presence of reciprocal changes in leads V1–3. Consider doing a posterior ECG in any patient with chest pain and a dominant R wave (R/S ratio > 1) in V2.

Emergency treatment of chest pain

- ABCDE approach: consider early oxygen and analgesia for pain
- Commence pulse oximetry and ECG monitoring
- Target oxygen therapy (if necessary) to achieve an arterial blood oxygen saturation of 94–98% (88–92% in the presence of chronic obstructive pulmonary disease [COPD])
- Secure IV access and request appropriate blood tests, e.g. full blood count, urea and electrolytes (U&Es), troponin, lipid profile, and blood glucose
- Perform a 12 lead ECG, regardless of the presumed cause of the pain

- Undertake a focused history: take a full chest pain history, including time of onset, duration, nature, exacerbating and relieving factors, and associated symptoms, plus enquiry regarding risk factors for cardiovascular and thromboembolic disease
- Request a chest X-ray: ensure prompt interpretation
- Place the patient in a comfortable position. This is usually a semi-recumbent position. If the patient is hypotensive or is feeling lightheaded, lie them flat
- Ensure appropriate help is called
- Identify and treat any underlying electrolyte abnormalities (hypokalaemia can complicate ACS)
- Identify and promptly treat complications, e.g. pulmonary oedema, cardiac arrhythmias
- Reassure patient

Initial treatment of ACS

- Assuming there is no definite allergy, administer aspirin (300 mg loading dose)
- Administer nitrates, e.g. buccal or sublingual (GTN), however for patients with ongoing pain consider early IV GTN infusion – this should be given in a monitored area and the dose titrated to the patient's symptoms and blood pressure. Patients with known aortic stenosis should not be given nitrates.
- Aim for oxygen saturations of 94–98% and administer oxygen accordingly
- Administer appropriate pain relief: it is important to render the patient pain-free as this reduces the stress on the myocardium; opiates, e.g. morphine or diamorphine IV, are usually used. There is usually no need to administer an antiemetic in the absence of nausea provided the drugs are given slowly and titrated to the patient's pain
- Patients with a STEMI (or new left bundle branch block): consider the need for early coronary reperfusion therapy (Box 13.1). This may necessitate transfer to another hospital
- The receiving unit will advise on which medications to administer prior to transfer, according to their local protocol
- Administer clopidogrel (300 mg loading dose) to all patients with suspected ACS, unless there is a specific contraindication (or significant bleeding risk)
- Consider low molecular weight heparin unless there is a significant bleeding risk (or other contraindication) or it is likely that a coronary angiogram is to be performed within 24 hours (in which case unfractionated heparin should be used)
- Consider glycoprotein IIb/IIIa receptor antagonist in high-risk patients with NSTEMI

Box 13.1 Coronary reperfusion therapy for STEMI

Gold standard reperfusion therapy is via percutaneous coronary intervention (PCI) and most trusts have access to a 24 hour service. Patients may be given high dose (600 mg) clopidogrel, or prasugrel, depending on trust protocols. Where PCI is not available, thrombolysis should be considered.

 Uncommon presentations

Sometimes ACS can present with pain in the jaw only. Patients with diabetes may present very atypically and sometimes even without pain, because of impaired cardiac innervation.

14 Management of abdominal pain

> **Definition:**
> - This is any serious acute intra-abdominal condition of less than 24 hours duration characterised by pain, tenderness, and muscular rigidity and for which emergency surgery must be considered
> - The term 'acute abdomen' is often used synonymously with acute peritonitis, which is defined as 'acute inflammation of the peritoneum which lines the abdominal cavity'

Incidence

- Abdominal pain is a very common problem in secondary care
- Whilst over 1000 causes exist >80% can be attributed to the following:
  - Non-specific abdominal pain (around 50% of cases)
  - Acute appendicitis: may be perforated
  - Acute cholecystitis
  - Acute diverticulitis: may be perforated
  - Small bowel obstruction
  - Acute pancreatitis
  - Upper gastrointestinal (gastric or duodenal) perforation
  - Ischaemic bowel: may be perforated
  - Perforated tumours (colonic)
  - Stercoral perforation (large bowel perforation secondary to constipation)

Medical Student Survival Skills: The Acutely Ill Patient, First Edition. Philip Jevon, Konnur Ramkumar, and Emma Jenkinson.
© 2020 John Wiley & Sons Ltd. Published 2020 by John Wiley & Sons Ltd.
Companion website: www.wiley.com/go/jevon/medicalstudent

Causes

- *Appendicitis*
  - Annually 60 000 cases
  - Lifetime risk of 7%
  - Death rate for perforated appendicitis 1.7% versus 0.3% for no perforation
  - Classic history of migratory right iliac fossa pain with anorexia
  - Atypical history dependent on position of appendix
    - Pelvic appendicitis: abdominal tenderness less marked
    - Retrocaecal appendicitis: tenderness marked in right flank
    - Pre/post-ileal appendicitis: diarrhoea may be a feature
- *Cholecystitis*
  - Acute inflammation of the gallbladder leading to marked pain in the right upper quadrant
  - Lifetime prevalence of 10%, of whom 80% have no symptoms
  - 1–3% of people with gallstones go on to develop cholecystitis
- *Diverticulitis*
  - Inflammation of diverticulae (acquired outpouchings of mucosa) commonly of the colon due to increased intraluminal pressure
  - Increased incidence with age; more common >50 years of age
  - Spectrum of presentation ranging from paracolic abscess to four-quadrant faecal peritonitis
- *Small bowel obstruction*
  - Obstruction of small bowel leading to copious bilious vomiting, colicky abdominal pain, and abdominal distension (late sign)
  - Common causes are abdominal wall herniae and adhesions secondary to previous surgery
  - Obstruction may lead to ischaemia/perforation of small bowel
- *Pancreatitis*
  - An inflammatory process with the potential to cause multiple organ failure
  - Commonly due to gallstones, alcohol, or idiopathic
  - Clinical signs such as left flank ecchymosis (Grey Turner's sign) and peri-umbilical ecchymosis (Cullen's sign) occur with haemorrhagic pancreatitis
  - Glasgow scoring on admission (Box 14.1) is important to stratify risk of multiple organ failure and to prompt high dependency unit (HDU) admission for monitoring

> **Box 14.1 Modified glasgow score for risk stratification of acute pancreatitis**
>
> Three or more positive criteria indicate severe pancreatitis necessitating HDU monitoring:
> - $PaO_2 < 8\,kPa$
> - Age > 55 years
> - White cell count > $15\,000 \times 10^9$
> - Corrected calcium < $2\,mmol\,l^{-1}$
> - Blood urea > $16\,mmol\,l^{-1}$
> - Enzymes: lactate dehydrogenase > $600\,IU\,l^{-1}$ or aspartate aminotransferase/alanine aminotransferase > $200\,IU\,l^{-1}$
> - Albumin < $32\,g\,l^{-1}$
> - Glucose > $10\,mmol\,l^{-1}$

Signs and symptoms

Symptoms may include:
- Severe generalised abdominal pain
- History may include a 'pop' at the point of rupture of a hollow viscus
- Anorexia, fever, vomiting
- Hiccups may occur with diaphragmatic irritation

Signs include:
- Explicit tenderness, guarding, rigidity in all quadrants of the abdomen
- Subtle maximal tenderness with or without a mass over the area of underlying pathology
- Abdominal distension
- Tachycardia, fever, hypotension
- Hypovolaemic/septic shock

Diagnosis

Diagnosis of a likely cause of acute abdomen lies with an accurate, focused history. Peritonitis is a clinical diagnosis but likely causes should be apparent from the history taken from the patient.

In addition to the presenting complaint, pay particular attention to systemic features such as weight loss, changes in bowel habit, previous surgery, alcohol intake, and concurrent medical problems such as atrial fibrillation and recent myocardial infarction.

ABCDE

- *Airway* – rarely affected
- *Breathing* – tachypnoea, shallow breathing, splinting of the diaphragm
- *Circulation* – tachycardia, hypotension, pallor, clammy, prolonged capillary refill time. In severe sepsis, warm peripheries with a bounding pulse may be present
- *Disability* – an altered level of consciousness is commonly due to sepsis, deranged blood sugar levels, or decreased cerebral perfusion due to extreme hypovolaemia
- *Exposure* – peripherally shut down, Cullen's sign/Grey Turner's sign with haemorrhagic pancreatitis

Investigations

- Routine bloods including full blood count, international normalised ratio, urea and electrolytes (U&Es), group and save cross match, amylase, C-reactive protein
- Urine dipstick +/– MC&S: note that the presence of blood may support a diagnosis of renal colic, the presence of white cells/nitrites may support a diagnosis of urinary tract infection, however these must be interpreted in the context of the history and examination findings. A positive urine dip does not exclude appendicitis, in fact the inflamed tip may irritate the bladder resulting resulting in the presence of white cells/blood.
- Erect chest X-ray (if perforation suspected)/abdominal X-ray (if bowel obstruction suspected)
- Arterial blood gas analysis
- 12 lead electrocardiogram (ECG)
- Computed tomography (CT) of the abdomen/pelvis
  Even when peritonitis is confirmed clinically, a CT scan can provide added information, such as the presence of metastatic disease, which can aid operative decision making.

 NB Intestinal obstruction and visceral perforation are the only indications for plain abdominal radiograph. The absence of pneumoperitoneum on an erect chest radiograph does not exclude visceral rupture.

Emergency treatment of abdominal pain

 NB Immediate management commonly focuses on resuscitating the patient, whilst starting definitive management and preparing the patient for the operating theatre where appropriate. When a patient is septic, management should include the 'Surviving Sepsis Campaign Bundle' (Box 14.2) and management of sepsis according to local protocol.

- ABCDE approach: consider early oxygen and analgesia (where appropriate)
- Commence pulse oximetry
- Target oxygen therapy (if necessary) to achieve an arterial blood oxygen saturation of 94–98% (88–92% in the presence of chronic obstructive pulmonary disease)
- Obtain wide bore IV access: commence IV fluids, e.g. crystalloids 30 ml kg^{-1}
- Where necessary, instigate management of sepsis including administration of IV antibiotics and blood cultures where appropriate (see Box 14.2).

Box 14.2 Surviving sepsis campaign bundle

To be completed within 3 hours:
- Measure lactate level
- Obtain blood cultures prior to administration of antibiotics
- Administer broad spectrum antibiotics
- Administer 30 ml kg^{-1} crystalloid for hypotension or lactate $\geq$ 4 mmol l^{-1}

To be completed within 6 hours:
- Apply vasopressors (for hypotension that does not respond to initial fluid resuscitation) to maintain a mean arterial pressure (MAP) $\geq$ 65 mmHg
- In the event of persistent arterial hypotension despite volume resuscitation (septic shock) or initial lactate $\geq$ 4 mmol l^{-1} (36 mg dl^{-1}):
  - Measure central venous pressure (CVP)[a]
  - Measure central venous oxygen saturation (ScvO$_2$)[a]
- Remeasure lactate if initial lactate was elevated[a]

[a] Targets for quantitative resuscitation included in the guidelines are a CVP of $\geq$ 8 mmHg; ScvO$_2$ of $\geq$ 70%, and normalisation of lactate.

- Administer IV broad-spectrum antibiotics, according to local protocol, if indicated
- Catheterise patients where there is hypotension/deranged renal function
- Administer appropriate analgesia, e.g. IV paracetamol, and IV opiates, e.g. morphine
- Consider nasogastric tube if the patient is vomiting
- Keep the patient nil by mouth
- Perform a 12 lead ECG to exclude a cardiac cause
- Reassess ABCDE

Early investigation and management

- Erect chest X-ray/abdominal X-ray
- Escalation to a senior surgical colleague
- Involvement of anaesthetic team if theatre is likely or there is severe pancreatitis
- Request a CT scan

 Uncommon presentations

Many rare causes of acute abdomen exist including torsion of the omentum, haematoma of the falciform ligament, mesenteroaxial gastric volvulus, and schistosomal peritonitis to name but a few. The approach to assessment of any acute abdomen is as in this chapter and should not be forgotten when rare pathology is suspected.

 Common interpretations and pitfalls

Consider non-surgical causes such as atypical pain from:
- Cardiac causes, e.g. acute myocardial infarction
- Respiratory causes, e.g. lower lobe pneumonia
- Gynaecological causes, e.g. pelvic inflammatory disease
- Endocrine causes, e.g. diabetic ketoacidosis
- Urological causes, e.g. referred pain from testicular torsion, ureteric stones

Management of acute ischaemic leg

G. R. Layton, G. Seyan, and I. Chukwulobelu

Manor Hospital, Walsall, UK

> **Definition:** Sudden reduction of blood flow to a limb that threatens the viability of a limb with previously adequate perfusion.

Background

- Onset is any period of time of less than 2 weeks
- The causes can be divided into three groups:
  - Thrombosis of a vessel with existing atherosclerotic plaque (60%)
  - Thromboembolism (30%)
  - Other (i.e. arterial dissection, trauma, iatrogenic injury) (10%)

> **NB** Most limb ischaemia is now due to acute thrombosis on a background of peripheral arterial disease. This can be more difficult to diagnose due to the development of collateral blood supply which attenuates the classic symptoms of acute ischaemia.

Incidence

- It is more common in the lower limb than the upper limb but either can be affected
  - Lower limb ischaemia affects 9–16 people per 100 000 per year
  - Upper limb ischaemia affects 1–3 people per 100 000 per year

Medical Student Survival Skills: The Acutely Ill Patient, First Edition. Philip Jevon, Konnur Ramkumar, and Emma Jenkinson.
© 2020 John Wiley & Sons Ltd. Published 2020 by John Wiley & Sons Ltd.
Companion website: www.wiley.com/go/jevon/medicalstudent

Morbidity and mortality

- Acute limb ischaemia carries a high morbidity and mortality
- It estimated that mortality due to acute ischaemia is as high as 22%
- It is estimated that 70–90% of limbs can be salvaged following acute limb ischaemia. However, many patients will require amputation which carries a high morbidity

Pathophysiology

There are two key mechanisms of action resulting in the development of acute limb ischaemia (Table 15.1).

- Thrombosis in situ
  - Plaque rupture in an atherosclerotic vessel resulting in the formation of a thrombus that occludes the vessel
- Thromboembolism
  - A thrombus forms away from the site of ischaemia and embolises into a limb where it becomes trapped within a vessel, resulting in occlusion
  - The commonest cause of embolism is atrial fibrillation; in these patients, the thrombus forms initially in the left atrium
  - Other causes of embolism include mural wall thrombosis after myocardial infarction and aneurysmal disease

Table 15.1 A comparison between an existing thrombosis and a sudden embolism

	Existing thrombosis	Embolism
Onset	Hours to days	Sudden
Severity	May be profound or may be less severe due to collaterals	Profound ischaemia
Embolic source	Will have risk factors for peripheral arterial disease	Usually atrial fibrillation. Less likely to have risk factors for peripheral arterial disease
Claudication history	Likely	Less likely

Signs and symptoms

Clinical presentation depends on the underlying pathology and time since onset (Table 15.2). The classic presentation of the six 'P's are often a late finding.

Table 15.2 Signs and prognosis of acute leg ischaemia

Time since onset	0–6 hours	6–12 hours	12 hours
Signs	Painful Dusky or white foot Neurosensory deficit, may be incomplete	Non-fixed mottling, blanches on pressure	Fixed mottling, does not blanch with pressure
Prognosis	Reversible	Partially reversible, dependent on underlying cause and coexisting disease	Irreversible

The classic presentation of an acutely ischaemic limb is also known as the six 'P's:

- **P**ale
- **P**ulseless
- **P**ainful
- **P**aralysis
- **P**araesthesia
- **P**erishingly cold

Diagnosis

- The purpose of assessment of patients with acute limb ischaemia is to consider:
  - Is the limb acutely ischaemic or is there an alternative cause?
  - Is this likely to be secondary to an embolic or thrombotic event?
  - Is the leg viable, threatened, or irreversibly ischaemic and therefore not salvageable?
- History will provide evidence of embolic source (acute onset or chronic), pre-existing peripheral arterial disease, or risk factors for atherosclerosis
- Examination of the cardiovascular system and neurovascular status of the limbs will also provide clues as to a patient's risk of acute ischaemia
- Diagnosis is largely clinical due to the presence of presenting signs and symptoms, including an inability to palpate peripheral pulses, and is supported by the finding of inadequate blood flow during examination with a hand-held Doppler ultrasound

Classification of acute limb ischaemia

The Rutherford (2009) classification is a clinical staging system used to objectively assess the severity of acute limb ischaemia (Table 15.3) and has been proposed as the basis for deciding between the various management options available.

Table 15.3 Grading system for acute limb ischaemia

	Capillary return	Motor	Sensory	Arterial Doppler signal	Venous Doppler signal
I Viable	–	–	–	–	–
IIa Threatened (salvageable if promptly treated)	Intact/ slow	Nil	Partial sensory deficit in digits only (or no deficit)	Often nil	–
IIb Threatened (salvageable with immediate intervention)	Slow/ absent	Partial paralysis	Partial sensory deficit in more than digits alone or complete deficit	Usually nil	–
III Irreversible (tissue loss or permanent nerve damage is inevitable despite intervention)	Absent and skin staining	Profound paralysis	Profound sensory deficit (anaesthetic)	Nil	Nil

Differential diagnosis

- *Compartment syndrome*: presents with severe pain and later, with neurosensory loss
- *Cerebrovascular accident*: limb may be pale, paralysed, or have paraesthesia but should not be painful. Doppler signals should be normal
- *Deep vein thrombosis*: limb may be warm, pink, swollen, and painful but should not exhibit neurovascular deficit. Arterial Doppler signals should be audible although venous Doppler signals may be abnormal
- *Hypovolaemic shock*: can present with pale, cool, pulseless limbs due to hypotension but this should be easy to differentiate through history and is likely to affect all limbs and not one in isolation
- *Acute compressive neuropathy*: can present with a paralysed limb. Doppler signals should be normal

 Common pitfalls and mistakes

A hand-held Doppler assessment of a suspected acutely ischaemic limb is essential. Pulses may be present but difficult to palpate. Alternatively, the absence of signal on Doppler suggests a diagnosis of limb ischaemia with the history and clinical examination confirming whether this is acute or chronic. Furthermore, the presence of weak but palpable pulses does not exclude ischaemia as a possible diagnosis. There may still be incomplete, and possibly critical, disruption of the blood supply.

ABCDE and SBAR

- *Airway*: unlikely to be affected
- *Breathing*: tachypnoea (due to acidosis from ischaemia)
- *Circulation*: irregularly irregular heart rate (from atrial fibrillation [AF], a possible source of embolism), tachycardia (due to non-rate-controlled AF, sepsis, or pain), prolonged capillary refill time in affected limb, or murmurs suggestive of valvular disease
- *Disability*: altered level of consciousness, e.g. confusion due to sepsis
- *Exposure*: dusky, white, or mottled limbs which may or may not blanch with digital pressure, absent peripheral pulses, and evidence of peripheral arterial disease, i.e. ulcers, trophic changes to skin
- *SBAR*: be clear when discussing your concerns with seniors. If you suspect acute ischaemia, this is a limb-threatening emergency requiring urgent senior review

NB
- A limb with sensorimotor deficit requires urgent assessment and intervention
- Fixed mottling and complete paralysis are signs of irreversible ischaemia and a non-viable limb

Immediate management of acute ischaemia

First line treatment
- Any patient with suspected acute ischaemia requires urgent admission to hospital
- Assess and treat the patient following the ABCDE approach
  - If the patient is showing any signs of septic shock, resuscitate the patient.

- Once acute limb ischaemia is recognised, call for help from senior colleagues
  - This should be your registrar within your own specialty. They will advise you on how to proceed but it is likely that they will advise you to call the vascular surgery team
- Administer analgesia
- Prepare the patient for possible emergency surgery
  - Keep the patient nil by mouth
  - IV access with IV fluids
  - Send a full set of blood tests including full blood count (FBC), urea and electrolytes (U&Es), liver function tests (LFTs), and a group and save (G&S)

NB A patient who is nil by mouth will require maintenance fluids. Furthermore, a patient with acute limb ischaemia will also be at risk of acute kidney injury due to rhabdomyolysis as the ischaemia progresses. Therefore IV fluids can help to optimise renal function by reducing the risk of pre-renal stresses on the kidneys such as hypovolaemia.

Surgical treatment
- If the occlusion is embolic, the options are surgical embolectomy or local intra-arterial thrombolysis
- If the occlusion is thrombotic, then the options are intra-arterial thrombolysis, angioplasty, or bypass surgery
- For patients in whom surgery is not in their best interests (for example, due to extremely high risk from anaesthesia), then palliative care alone may be offered

NB Patients who develop acute limb ischaemia are likely to have a history of cardiovascular co-morbidities such as a previous stroke or atrial fibrillation. Therefore, many patients may be taking antiplatelet therapy (such as clopidogrel) or anticoagulation (such as warfarin). If a patient is to undergo intra-arterial thrombolysis or surgery it is important that their clotting profile is assessed and that emergency reversal of this is considered if appropriate. Reversing coagulopathy is dependent on the anticoagulant agent but is often done with vitamin K or human prothrombin complex (synthetic clotting factors). *The decision to reverse coagulopathy should be made by a senior doctor such as your registrar so always seek their advice early.*

Investigations

- Full set of acute admission bloods including FBC, U&Es, LFTs, bone profile, C-reactive protein, G&S, and clotting profile
- Arterial blood gas analysis
- 12 lead electrocardiogram
- Chest X-ray
- Bedside Doppler

16 Management of acute kidney injury

Gareth Lodwick

New Cross Hospital, Wolverhampton, UK

> **Definition:** Acute deterioration in renal function, including loss of fluid, and electrolyte and acid–base homeostasis.

Incidence

- Up to 5% all hospital admissions in UK are due to acute kidney injury (AKI)
- Incidence increases with age

Deaths associated with AKI

- Mortality ranges from 10% to 80%
- There is 10% mortality in uncomplicated AKI
- There is up to 80% mortality if renal replacement therapy is required

Causes

Causes include:
- Renal hypoperfusion causing ischaemia leading to acute tubular necrosis (ATN)
  - Sepsis
  - Blood loss
  - Myocardial depression
- Nephrotoxic medications – (gentamicin, non-steroidal anti-inflammatory drugs, angiotensin-converting enzyme inhibitors, diuretics, etc.)
- Urinary tract obstruction
  - Urinary retention

Medical Student Survival Skills: The Acutely Ill Patient, First Edition. Philip Jevon, Konnur Ramkumar, and Emma Jenkinson.
© 2020 John Wiley & Sons Ltd. Published 2020 by John Wiley & Sons Ltd.
Companion website: www.wiley.com/go/jevon/medicalstudent

- Toxic ATN
  - Rhabdomyolysis
  - Contrast nephropathy
- Structural abnormalities
  - Renovascular occlusion
  - Small vessel occlusion
- Acute glomerulonephritis/vasculitis
  - Goodpasture's syndrome
  - Antineutrophil cytoplasmic antibody (ANCA) positive glomerulonephritis
  - Idiopathic crescentic glomerulonephritis
- Interstitial nephritis
  - Infections
- Myeloma

Pathophysiology

- Acute tubular necrosis occurs following reduction in blood supply causing ischaemic injury
- Afferent arteriolar vasoconstriction occurs due to vasoconstrictors (endothelin) and reduced dilators (nitric oxide)
- This causes redistribution of blood and hypoxic injury to the kidney
- Cell necrosis occurs leading to formation of casts that block the flow of urine

Signs and symptoms

Signs and symptoms may include:
- Fatigue
- Confusion
- Anorexia
- Headache
- Nausea and vomiting
- Flank pain
- Cardiac arrhythmias – due to the raised potassium level

Investigations

- Blood tests: urea and electolytes (U&Es), full blood count (FBC), liver function tests (LFTs), clotting, creatine kinase (CK), C-reactive protein (CRP), phosphate, calcium, and magnesium

- Blood gases: for potassium and acid–base balance
- ECG: hyperkalaemia changes (Box 16.1)
- Urine dipstick
- Urine proteins
- Urgent ultrasound of renal tract: to exclude obstruction
- Chest X-ray: pulmonary oedema (upper lobe diversion, Kerly's B lines, increased lung markings, pleural effusions)
- If cause is unclear or there are signs of vasculitis (nosebleeds or rashes):
  - Immunoglobulins, electrophoresis, autoantibodies (antinuclear antibodies, ANCA, anti-dsDNA, antiglomerular basement membrane)
  - Consider biopsy – needs renal opinion

Box 16.1 ECG changes with hyperkalemia

- Tall tented T waves
- Small or absent P waves
- Widened QRS
- Sine wave pattern
- Asystole

Diagnosis

- Reduction in estimated glomerular filtration rate (GFR) or raised creatinine as classified by RIFLE criteria (Box 16.2)
- Acute versus chronic:
  - Co-morbidity leading to chronic failure
  - Previous blood tests

Box 16.2 Rifle criteria from the acute dialysis quality initiative

- **R**isk: GFR drop > 25%, creatinine ×1.5, or < 0.5 ml kg h^{-1} urine for 6 hours
- **I**njury: GFR drop > 50%, creatinine ×2, or < 0.5 ml kg h^{-1} urine for 12 hours
- **F**ailure: GFR drop > 75%, creatinine ×3, or > 355 µmol l^{-1} (> 44 increase) or < 0.3 ml kg^{-1}h^{-1} urine for 24 hours
- **L**oss: persistent AKI or complete loss of renal function for more than 4 weeks
- **E**nd stage renal disease: need for renal replacement therapy for 3 months

- Is urinary tract obstruction present:
  - Pain, i.e. renal stones
  - Lower urinary tract symptoms (urinary retention, BPH)
  - Are they oliguric: $<0.5\,ml\,kg^{-1}\,h^{-1}$

Initial treatment

- Assess and treat the patient following the ABCDE approach
- Optimise fluid balance to maintain normal blood pressure for individual
  - Avoid hypovolaemia/overload
- Treat any underlying sepsis or shock
- Urgent ECG and blood potassium check (use a venous blood gas to obtain a rapid sample whilst laboratory values are awaited): treat hyperkalaemia if present
- Stop all nephrotoxic medications
- Maintain strict fluid balance monitoring; insert urinary catheter if necessary
- Undertake investigations (see earlier)
- Maintain nutrition
- Obtain senior support for ongoing management
- Consider renal replacement therapy, and intensive treatment unit/high dependency unit referral

> **NB** Indications for urgent renal replacement therapy include:
> - Severe uraemia (encephalopathy, vomiting, and urea $>60\,mmol\,l^{-1}$)
> - Persistent hyperkalaemia: $>7\,mmol\,l^{-1}$, ECG changes, or >6.5 and unresponsive to treatment
> - Severe metabolic acidosis pH 7.2 or base excess <10, i.e. failure to compensate
> - Uraemic pericarditis
> - Refractory pulmonary oedema

Treatment of associated conditions

- *Hyperkalaemia*
  - IV calcium – 10 ml 10% calcium gluconate for cardioprotection
  - IV insulin and dextrose – 10 units actrapid in 50 ml 50% glucose over 30 minutes (or as per local protocol) – recheck glucose after 30 minutes
  - Salbutamol nebuliser 5 mg

- – Consider calcium resonium 15 g/8 h to bind K+ in the gastointestinal tract with a slower mechanism of action
  - – Haemofiltration
- *Pulmonary oedema*
  - – Sit up, high-flow oxygen
  - – Vasodilators (e.g. morphine 2.5 mg)
  - – Furosemide (may need higher doses in renal failure – if unsure consult senior)
  - – Haemofiltration
  - – Consider continuous positive airway pressure and IV nitrates infusion
- Bleeding – raised urea can lead to impaired clotting
  - – Replace fluids
  - – Fresh frozen plasma and platelets – discuss with haematologists

 Common misinterpretations and pitfalls

- Assuming dehydration as cause and failure to assess for obstruction or rarer causes
- Failure to recheck U&Es including potassium after treatment to check response

SBAR approach

After basic tests are done or if the patient meets the criteria for urgent renal replacement therapy, contact senior support using the framework below.

- **S**ituation: You have a patient with acute kidney injury – *I have a 63-year-old man with acute kidney injury admitted with confusion*
- **B**ackground: Mention the patient's background medical problems and initial test results – *He has a background of asthma and had a recent flu-like illness, his estimated GFR is 30 (down from >90) and creatinine is 200. He is acidotic on gas with a normal lactate and potassium level of 4.9*
- **A**ssessment: Detail the assessment you have made, including important findings on investigations, what you think may be causing it and what treatment you have started – *He is mildly confused with an otherwise unremarkable examination apart from appearing dehydrated. His urine output is reduced as well. I believe he is dehydrated and this has caused his AKI, I have therefore sent off for blood tests, and started IV fluid replacement and fluid balance monitoring*

- **R**ecommendation: What you would like advice on, i.e. do you need help finding the diagnosis or with the next stages of treatment or do you feel the patient warrants renal replacement therapy and this needs to be arranged? – *I would like you to review him please and advise me on investigations I have missed or if he needs monitoring in a more intensive environment*

 Uncommon presentations

Patients who present following falls and long lies on the floor have a chance of rhabdomylosis causing the AKI.

OSCE Key Learning Points

✔ Diagnosis and recognition of blood test results
✔ Ensure check potassium and ECG
✔ Consider indications for renal replacement
✔ SBAR call for senior support

Management of the unconscious patient

17

Background

- Loss of consciousness is a common presentation of the acutely unwell patient
- There are multiple differential diagnoses
- Initial management is straightforward and involves an ABCDE approach
- Ultimate diagnosis and treatment may be complex

Pathophysiology

- There are multiple ways of classifying the causes of impaired consciousness
- Causes can be categorised according to the systems affected (Box 17.1)
- Causes can be described using a 'surgical sieve' (Box 17.2)

Box 17.1 Causes of reduced consciousness according to systems

- *Airway*: airway obstruction causing hypoxia
- *Breathing*: impaired oxygenation (hypoxia) or ventilation (hypercarbia)
- *Cardiovascular*: impaired cerebral perfusion due to shock
- *Disability*: primary neurological causes
- *Exposure*: hypothermia, hypoglycaemia, toxins

Medical Student Survival Skills: The Acutely Ill Patient, First Edition. Philip Jevon, Konnur Ramkumar, and Emma Jenkinson.
© 2020 John Wiley & Sons Ltd. Published 2020 by John Wiley & Sons Ltd.
Companion website: www.wiley.com/go/jevon/medicalstudent

Box 17.2 Surgical sieve of causes of unconsciousness

- *Vascular*: e.g. stroke, subarachnoid haemorrhage
- *Infective*: e.g. meningitis, encephalitis, abscesses
- *Autoimmune*: e.g. cerebral lupus
- *Traumatic*: e.g. contusions, haematoma
- *Neoplastic*: e.g. brain tumours
- *Degenerative*: e.g. dementia
- *Metabolic*: e.g. hypoglycaemia, hypercapnia, hyponatraemia, encephalopathy
- *Environmental*: e.g. drugs/toxins (including withdrawal of drugs, e.g. alcohol)
- *Congenital*: e.g. epilepsy
- *Psychiatric*: e.g. pseudoseizures, catatonia, functional loss of consciousness

Emergency treatment

Assuming the patient is not in cardiac arrest:

- Follow an ABCDE approach
- Request monitoring, e.g. blood pressure, pulse oximetry, and electro-cardiogram (ECG) as soon as possible

NB Correction of ABCDE problems may be sufficient to restore consciousness.

Airway assessment

- Perform head till/chin lift to open and clear airway. Relieve any obstruction with manual manoeuvres or adjuncts. Utilise suction if necessary
- Call for senior/anaesthetic input early if any airway problems are identified
- Administer oxygen 15l via a non-rebreathe oxygen mask. Target oxygen therapy to achieve an arterial blood oxygen saturation of 94–98% (88–92% in the presence of chronic obstructive pulmonary disease)
- Consider lateral position (recovery position)

NB Do not forget to consider immobilisation of the cervical spine if there is any possibility of head trauma.

Breathing assessment

- Perform respiratory assessment (inspection, palpation, and auscultation)
- In particular, assess breathing: respiratory rate and pattern of breathing (Cheyne–Stokes, Kussmaul?)
- Check oxygen saturations
- Perform arterial blood gas analysis. The presence of hypercapnia implies that ventilatory support may be required so seek early senior/specialist advice
- Monitor oxygen delivery
- Recheck airway patency

Circulation assessment

- Check pulse: rate (normal, fast, or slow) and rhythm (regular or irregular)
- Check for signs of hypoperfusion, including hypotension or delayed capillary refill and consider early fluid bolus
- Check ECG monitor: interpret ECG rhythm
- Check 12 lead ECG for arrhythmias or ischaemia and treat accordingly
- Perform IV access

Disability assessment

- Assess level of consciousness using AVPU (Box 17.3)
- Check size of pupils – normal, pinpoint, or dilated
- Check for pupillary response to light and accommodation; check consensual reaction
- Look for obvious lateralising signs and focal neurology or signs
- Check blood sugar (and correct accordingly)

Box 17.3 AVPU Scale

- **A**lert
- Responds to **V**oice
- Responds to **P**ain
- **U**nresponsive

 Common misinterpretations and pitfalls

Hypoglycaemia is a common cause of unconsciousness. Do not forget bedside blood sugar assessment.

Exposure

- Check for external signs of injury, e.g. head injury
- Check for signs of IV drug use
- Check for evidence of alcohol use
- Check environmental factors, e.g. temperature; rewarm if necessary

Formal assessment of conscious level

Following initial assessment, the Glasgow coma score (Box 17.4) should be determined.

Box 17.4 Glasgow coma score (GCS)		
Eyes (E)	Spontaneous	4
	To verbal stimulus	3
	To pain	2
	None	1
Verbal (V)	Orientated	5
	Confused speech	4
	Inappropriate words	3
	Incomprehensible noises	2
	None	1
Motor (M)	Obeys commands	6
	Localises pain	5
	Withdraws from pain	4
	Abnormal flexion	3
	Abnormal extension	2
	None	1

- A GCS of ≤8 indicates a patient's inability to protect their airway so senior support should be sought early for these patients

History taking

- Once the patient has been stabilised take a *focused* history
- This may require information from ambulance or ward staff, or relatives
- Ask about previously medical illness and drug history
- Ask about events leading up to the illness (e.g. fevers, trauma)

- Ask about alcohol and recreational drug use
- Ask about psychiatric history
- Ask about environmental factors (e.g. carbon monoxide)

Additional investigations

- Blood gas sample (Box 17.5)
- Laboratory blood samples (for inflammatory markers, electrolytes, etc.)
- Computed tomography (CT) head scan (if suspecting intracranial pathology)
- Magnetic resonance imaging scan
- Alcohol or drug levels (urine and serum samples)
- Lumbar puncture (if infection or subarachnoid haemorrhage are suspected)
- Electroencephalogram (if status epilepticus suspected)
- Serum ammonia levels (if encephalopathy suspected)

Box 17.5 Blood gases

Most blood gas machines will provide the following useful parameters:

- PO_2 (exclude hypoxia)
- PCO_2 (exclude hypercarbia)
- Haemoglobin (exclude profound anaemia)
- Carboxyhaemaglobin (exclude carbon monoxide poisoning)
- Electrolytes (exclude hyponatraemia, hypocalcaemia)
- pH/bicarbonate
- Lactate (may be elevated in sepsis or severe shock)
- Glucose

Specific management of common causes of impaired consciousness

- Stabilisation of ABCDE regardless of cause
- Do not forget to consider early airway and ventilatory support in patients with a reduced conscious level

Acute alcohol intoxication
- Treatment is largely supportive

- Patient is ideally nursed in the lateral position
- Intravenous fluids can support blood pressure and hasten recovery
- Airway and ventilatory support is occasionally required

Alcohol-related encephalopathy

- Administer vitamins (usually in the form of Pabrinex) immediately
- Administer 5% dextrose *after* vitamins have been given
- Involve seniors/specialists early

Alcohol withdrawal seizures

- Give intravenous benzodiazepines – large doses may be required
- Give Pabrinex early
- Correct blood sugar/electrolytes

Epileptic seizures

- Check blood sugar and electrolytes
- Follow National Institute for Health and Care Excellence (NICE) guidance on the management of seizures (www.nice.org.uk)
- Seek early senior support in case rapid sequence induction is required

Opiate overdose

- Naloxone can be used as a reversal agent
- Usually start with 400 µg IV *plus* a 400 µg IM dose
- Naloxone has a short half-life, and infusion may be required
- Caution in chronic opiate use as naloxone can precipitate withdrawal symptoms and aggressive behaviour

Benzodiazepine overdose

- Flumazenil can be used as a reversal agent but with extreme caution
- It is usually safer to manage the patient supportively

Meningitis/encephalitis

- Early antibiotics (usually ceftriaxone) and/or antivirals (usually aciclovir)
- Consider administration of steroids (dexamethasone)
- Consider loading with phenytoin or levetiracetam if there is seizure activity

Traumatic brain injury

- Seek early neurosurgical advice
- Institute early brain protection (optimise oxygenation/ventilation, manage patient in 30° head-up position, optimise fluid balance, etc.)

Space-occupying lesions

- Give dexamethasone
- Seek early specialist advice
- Consider loading with phenytoin or levetiracetam if there is seizure activity

Stroke

- Seek early specialist advice; may be suitable for thrombolysis
- See Chapter 12

Subarachnoid haemorrhage

- If CT confirms diagnosis, discuss with neurosurgeons
- If CT is normal, lumbar puncture should be performed at 12 hours
- Control blood pressure (usually using nimodipine)

 Common misinterpretations and pitfalls

Remember to exclude 'simple' treatable causes of unconsciousness, e.g. hypoxia, hypercapnia, profound bradycardia, shock, hypoglycaemia, and opiate administration.

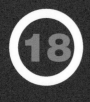

Management of upper gastrointestinal bleed

G. S. Seyan and I. Chukwulobelu

Manor Hospital, Walsall, UK

> **Definition:** An upper gastrointestinal bleed (UGIB) is bleeding that originates proximal to the ligament of Treitz, i.e. from the nasopharynx, oesophagus, stomach, or duodenum

Causes

- Peptic ulcer disease – bleeds from duodenal ulcers are more common than gastric ulcers
- Variceal bleed – oesophageal or gastric varices secondary to chronic portal hypertension
- Mallory–Weiss syndrome – oesophageal tear following vomiting
- Malignancy – oesophageal or gastric malignancy
- Drugs – non-steroidal anti-inflammatory drugs (NSAIDs), steroids, anticoagulants, and selective serotonin reuptake inhibitors (SSRIs)
- Other – gastritis, duodenitis, and oesophagitis

 NB In about 20% of cases, endoscopy does not reveal the source of bleeding.

Medical Student Survival Skills: The Acutely Ill Patient, First Edition. Philip Jevon, Konnur Ramkumar, and Emma Jenkinson.
© 2020 John Wiley & Sons Ltd. Published 2020 by John Wiley & Sons Ltd.
Companion website: www.wiley.com/go/jevon/medicalstudent

Incidence

- A common, life-threatening medical emergency affecting 1:1000 adults per year
- It is associated with an in-hospital mortality of 10%; mortality is highest in the over 60s and with variceal bleeds (Box 18.1)

Box 18.1 Poor prognostic indicators

- Age >60 years
- Two or more co-morbidities
- Chronic liver disease
- Features of shock
- Hospital in-patient at time of bleed

Risk factors

- Drugs (NSAIDs, steroids, anticoagulants, SSRIs)
- Portal hypertension – the most common causes are cirrhosis (UK) and schistosomiasis (worldwide)
- Previous history of upper gastrointestinal bleed
- Alcohol excess
- *Helicobacter pylori* infection

Symptoms and signs

- Haematemesis – vomiting of blood from upper gastrointestinal (GI) tract
  - Fresh red blood – suggests active bleeding
  - 'Coffee ground' – vomiting of altered, partly digested blood
- Melaena – passing of sticky, black, tarry stools
- Hypovolaemic shock and collapse
- Syncope and postural hypotension
- Chronic UGIB may present with symptoms and signs of iron deficiency anaemia, e.g. fatigue, angina, shortness of breath, altered bowel habit, and positive faecal occult blood test
- Haematochezia – passage of fresh or altered blood per rectum, an uncommon presentation of a profuse upper GI bleed (Table 18.1)

NB Be Aware!

- Evidence of postural hypotension is an indicator of hypovolaemic shock and can be an early sign
- Elderly patients have less physiological reserve and will decompensate early
- Young patients may not demonstrate signs of shock until a large volume loss occurs

ABCDE approach to examination and initial management

Table 18.1 ABCDE approach to the examination and initial management of UGIBs

	Examine	Measure/monitor	Treat/intervention	Investigations
Airway	Assess for sounds of airway obstruction or compromise	O_2 saturations Capnography	Suction may clear upper airway Simple airway adjuncts if reduced Glasgow coma score (GCS) Contact anaesthetist if airway compromise (GCS <8)	
Breathing	Inspect, palpate, percuss, and auscultate May have features of aspiration	O_2 saturations – may be hypoxic with large bleed Respiratory rate – may be tachypnoeic	High-flow oxygen (15 l min⁻¹) via non-rebreathe mask	Arterial blood gas (ABG) to assess for respiratory failure
Circulation	Inspect, palpate, and auscultate Assess capillary refill and check jugular venous pressure – may be peripherally prolonged and low	Heart rate – likely to be tachycardic Blood pressure (BP) – likely to be hypotensive and have postural hypotension Urine output – may be reduced	Secure IV access – two large bore cannulas Consider bolus fluids if hypotensive – e.g. 500 ml crystalloid stat; if actively bleeding, aim at systolic BP of >90 mmHg Catheterise and monitor urine output – aim to >0.5 ml kg⁻¹ h⁻¹	Urgent bloods – full blood count, urea and electrolytes (U&Es), liver function tests (LFTs), clotting, fibrinogen, group and save, cross match (2–4 units) ABG/venous blood gas – rapid haemoglobin value

(Continued)

Table 18.1 (Continued)

	Examine	Measure/monitor	Treat/intervention	Investigations
				Consider chest X-ray if signs of aspiration or bowel perforation
				Consider O-negative blood if massive blood loss
Disability	Assess pupil size and response Assess for any features of hepatic encephalopathy	Assess GCS Blood glucose	Appropriate analgesia if required	
Exposure	Assess for signs of chronic liver disease Abdominal examination – may have tenderness Digital rectal examination – may have melaena Check temperature		If signs of chronic liver disease and portal hypertension, then consider terlipressin Keep nil by mouth	Consider abdominal imaging if indicated

NB Be Aware!
- Monitor observations (BP, pulse, respiratory rate, and oxygen saturations every 15 minutes in the initial stages)
- Keep patient nil by mouth – they are likely to require endoscopy
- Use O-negative blood if there is massive blood loss
- Avoid dextrose solutions for resuscitation

Further treatment

- Calculate the Blatchford score and involve seniors (SBAR)
- Liaise with the endoscopy team once the patient has been resuscitated and stabilised
- Stop NSAIDs, diuretics, antihypertensives, and anticoagulants
- Repeat fluid boluses as required to keep systolic BP > 90 mmHg

- In patients with cardiac or renal disease, discuss with seniors about central pressure monitoring and high dependency unit (HDU) care
- Transfuse and aim for a haemoglobin of >8 g dl⁻¹
- Correct any coagulopathy before endoscopy
  - Reverse warfarin using 5–10 mg of vitamin K and prothrombin complex concentrates (e.g. Beriplex) if actively bleeding
  - If on dabigatran consider the use of idarucizumab for reversal
  - If on apixaban or rivaroxaban discuss reversal with haematology staff
  - If platelets are <50 and patient is actively bleeding then organise platelet transfusion
  - If fibrinogen is <1 g l⁻¹, contact haematologist department for advice
- Proton pump inhibitors (PPIs) should be started if there is a strong suspicion of peptic ulcer disease *and* if endoscopy is not available within 24 hours, otherwise await endoscopy before starting PPIs
  - When starting PPI therapy, give 80 mg omeprazole IV as a bolus followed by an IV infusion at 8 mg h⁻¹. PPI therapy improves outcomes post endoscopy
- If there are clinical features of portal hypertension and a variceal bleed is suspected, give 2 mg terlipressin and antibiotics in accordance with your trust guidelines (e.g. Tazocin)
- Consider assessment for *H. pylori* and eradication
- Endoscopy allows differentiation between different causes of bleeding and offers an opportunity for intervention
- Consider intensive treatment unit (ITU)/HDU setting if patient requires intubation or organ support; involve ITU early if patient is deteriorating or at high risk

NB Be Aware!
- The priority is to replace volume loss and restore BP – endoscopy is indicated once the patient has been resuscitated and stabilised
- Take a full drug history, including new oral anticoagulants, e.g. dabigatran, apixaban, and rivaroxaban

NB Your hospital trust's major haemorrhage protocol will provide advice on blood products.

Assessment of chronic liver disease in the emergency setting

In an unstable patient it may not possible to take a comprehensive history or perform a detailed examination but some targeted questions and examinations may indicate a patient with liver disease:

History

- Alcohol excess, chronic hepatitis, IV drug use, previous bleeds

Examination

- Signs of chronic liver disease, e.g. spider naevi, bruising, ascites, jaundice, palmar erythema, caput medusae, clubbing, gynaecomastia, encephalopathy

Blood tests

- Deranged LFTs, low albumin, thrombocytopenia, raised prothrombin time

Endoscopy and surgical intervention

- Endoscopy allows for the diagnosis of a bleed and its intervention
- Bleeding vessel or ulcer
  - Endoscopic adrenaline injection, thermal coagulation or clipping
  - If this fails, then surgical intervention, i.e. direct ligation is likely to be required
- Variceal bleed
  - Endoscopic banding, sclerotherapy, or adrenaline injections
  - If this fails, then surgical intervention, i.e. balloon tamponade (Sengstaken–Blakemore tube) or transjugular intrahepatic portosystemic shunt (TIPSS) may be required

Indications for surgical intervention

- Rebleeding, despite endoscopic interventions
- Exsanguinating haemorrhage or uncontrollable bleeding at endoscopy
- Special situations – e.g. rare blood group, refusing transfusion
- Initial Rockall score ≥3 or final score >6
- Bowel perforation

Assessment of risk

Two scoring systems are routinely use in the UK – the Blatchford score and Rockall score.

- The Blatchford risk score (Table 18.2) should be calculated on admission; it is used to predict the need for medical intervention, i.e. transfusion, endoscopic therapy, or surgery
  - A Blatchford score of zero suggests the patient may be suitable for discharge with out-patient endoscopy
- The Rockall score (Table 18.3) should be calculated after endoscopy and predicts the risk of rebleeding and mortality
- The Blatchford and Rockall scores should be calculated in all UGIBs.

Table 18.2 The Blatchford score

Admission parameter	Score value
Urea (mg dl⁻¹)	
≥6.5 to <8.0	2
≥8.0 to <10.0	3
≥10.0 to <25.0	4
≥25.0	6
Haemoglobin (g dl⁻¹)	
Men	
≥12.0 to <13.0	1
≥10.0 to <12.0	3
<10.0	6
Women	
≥10.0 to <12.0	1
<10.0	6
Systolic BP (mmHg)	
100 to 109	1
90 to 99	2
<90	3
Other parameters	
Pulse >100 bpm	1
Melaena at presentation	1
Syncope	2
Hepatic disease	2
Cardiac failure	2

Source: Blatchford et al. (2000).

Table 18.3 The Rockall score with corresponding mortality rate

Variable	Score 0	Score 1	Score 2	Score 3
Age (years)	<60	60–79	>80	
Co-morbidity	Nil major		Congestive heart failure Ischaemic heart disease	Renal failure Liver disease Metastatic cancer
Shock	No shock	Pulse >100 bpm	Systolic BP <100 mmHg	
Source of bleeding	Mallory–Weiss tear	All other diagnoses, e.g. oesophagitis, gastritis, peptic ulcer disease, varices	Malignancy	
Stigmata of recent bleeding	None		Adherent clot, spurting vessel	

Rockall score	Mortality (%)
0	0
1	0
2	0.2
3	3
4	5.3
5	11
6	17
7	27
8	41

Source: Rockall et al. (1996)

19 Management of diabetic ketoacidosis

> **Definition:** Diabetic ketoacidosis (DKA) is an acute complication of diabetes typically characterised by hyperglycaemia, ketone body formation, and metabolic acidosis.

 NB DKA can be life-threatening; if untreated coma and death will occur.

Prognosis

- DKA remains a major contributor to morbidity and mortality in diabetes
- Mortality rates: 5–10%, even as high as 20% in the elderly
- Mortality is usually due to an underlying morbidity, e.g. sepsis or acute coronary syndrome
- It is the commonest cause of death in young persons with diabetes

 NB Delays in diagnosis and errors in management can lead to death.

Incidence

- DKA accounted for nearly 8400 hospital admissions in England in 2004/2005
- It is usually associated with new cases of type 1 diabetes. It can also occur in type 2 diabetes, particularly in African-American and ethnic minorities, particularly when severe stress, e.g. sepsis or trauma, is present

Medical Student Survival Skills: The Acutely Ill Patient, First Edition. Philip Jevon, Konnur Ramkumar, and Emma Jenkinson.
© 2020 John Wiley & Sons Ltd. Published 2020 by John Wiley & Sons Ltd.
Companion website: www.wiley.com/go/jevon/medicalstudent

Pathophysiology

- Severe insulin deficiency (partial or complete), together with elevated levels of circulating catecholamines and other stress hormones, lead to increased glucose production in the liver and impaired glucose uptake in the tissues
- There is increased lipolysis (fat breakdown), and ketone bodies are produced leading to metabolic acidosis
- Hyperglycaemia causes a profound osmotic diuresis that leads to dehydration and loss of electrolytes, particularly sodium and potassium. The loss of potassium is further exacerbated by metabolic acidosis and vomiting

Causes

Causes of DKA include:
- Infection (30–50%): usually urinary tract infection or pneumonia
- Newly presenting type 1 diabetes (10–20%)
- Errors with insulin administration (15–30%): e.g. giving the wrong dose of insulin, omitting dose(s), or failing to increase the dose during episodes of illness
- Intercurrent illnesses: e.g. surgery, trauma, myocardial ischaemia, pancreatitis
- Miscellaneous (5%): e.g. drugs or alcohol misuse
- Unknown (40%)

Signs and symptoms

NB The presentation of DKA is usually within 24 hours, although symptoms may be present for several days before ketoacidosis develops.

Clinical features of DKA include:
- Polyuria – due to osmotic diuresis
- Polydipsia – due to osmotic diuresis
- Weight loss – due to catabolism and dehydration
- Generalised weakness

- Fruity odour on the breath – sometimes described as a pear drop or a nail varnish type of smell; this is due to ketones being excreted via the lungs
- Kussmaul's respirations – rapid deep breathing due to metabolic acidosis
- Nausea and vomiting (present in 50–80% of patients)
- Abdominal pain (present in about 30% of cases)
- Coma (present in 10% of cases)

Investigations

Investigations that should be undertaken include:
- Bedside assessment of blood glucose and blood ketones
- Routine bloods: urea and electrolytes (U&Es), full blood count, glucose and bicarbonate
- Arterial blood gas analysis
- Urinalysis to detect ketonuria
- Infection screen: blood and urine cultures, C-reactive protein (CRP) and chest X-ray
- ECG

Diagnosis

- Blood glucose > 13.8 mmol l^{-1}
- pH < 7.30
- Serum bicarbonate < 18 mmol l^{-1}
- Anion gap > 10
- Ketonaemia

Emergency treatment of DKA

OSCE Key Learning Points

✔ The treatment of DKA involves careful clinical evaluation, correction of metabolic abnormalities, identification and treatment of precipitating and co-morbid conditions, appropriate long-term treatment of diabetes, and plans to prevent recurrence

- ABCDE approach
- Establish blood pressure, electrocardiogram (ECG), and pulse oximetry monitoring
- Ensure the patient has a clear airway – if the patient has an altered conscious level, their airway is at risk. Place in recovery position if necessary
- Consider inserting a basic airway device, e.g. oropharyngeal airway, if the patient is unconscious. Consider the need for tracheal intubation
- Administer high-flow oxygen using a non-rebreathe mask. Establish oxygen saturation monitoring using a pulse oximeter
- Check arterial blood gases
- Insert a wide bore IV cannula (e.g. 14G)
- Commence IV fluids: 1000 ml of 0.9% normal saline in the first hour, followed by 500 ml h^{-1} in the next 2–3 hours. It is usual to replace the fluid deficit (5–8 l in DKA) over a period of 24 hours. The actual rate of fluid administration will depend on the patient's clinical status, e.g. in shock, the infusion rate will need to be increased. Change to 0.45% normal saline if the plasma sodium is > 150 mmol l^{-1}. The intracellular water deficit needs to be replaced using a dextrose (10%) and not a saline solution; this is done once the blood glucose levels are < 15 mmol

NB It is important to avoid rapid IV infusion in patients with cardiovascular compromise and in young patients for whom there is a risk of cerebral oedema developing.

- Establish continuous ECG monitoring: electrolyte abnormalities, particularly hypokalaemia, can cause life-threatening cardiac arrhythmias
- Monitor plasma glucose levels regularly, initially at least hourly
- Commence low-dose insulin (0.1 unit/kg/hr) via IV infusion (6 units h^{-1}) (other routes are possible for insulin administration, e.g. subcutaneous); once the blood sugar is < 15 mmol l^{-1}, reduce the insulin infusion to 4 units h^{-1} and replace the saline infusion with 10% dextrose
- Administer potassium 20 mmol h^{-1} via a potassium chloride solution unless the plasma potassium is > 5.5 mmol; note that although total body potassium is low, plasma potassium levels may be normal, low, or high
- Closely monitor plasma potassium levels (optimal range is 4–5 mmol l^{-1})
- If plasma pH is < 7, administer sodium bicarbonate 1.4% 500 ml over 30 minutes

- Consider inserting a nasogastric tube if the patient has an impaired conscious level, because of the risk of gastroparesis, vomiting/regurgitation of gastric contents, and aspiration
- Insert a urinary catheter and closely monitor urine output
- Consider broad-spectrum antibiotics if an infection is suspected; pyrexia is rarely present and an increase in white cell count could just be due to ketonaemia
- Consider inserting a central venous catheter to monitor central venous pressure (e.g. in critical illness)
- Closely monitor the patient's vital signs, fluid balance, blood glucose, blood ketones, arterial blood gases, and U&Es
- Involve the diabetes team at the earliest opportunity, e.g. making the decision to stop continuous IV infusion of insulin to subcutaneous injections of insulin is best made by senior experienced medical staff
- Appropriate on-going care is essential

Complications

Complications of DKA include:
- Cerebral oedema: causes include rapid reduction of blood glucose and use of hypotonic fluids and/or bicarbonate
- Acute respiratory distress syndrome
- Deep vein thrombosis and pulmonary embolism (hyperglycaemia causes a hypercoagulable state)
- Acute circulatory failure: due to rapid IV infusion of fluids

Hyperosmolar non-ketotic coma

- Hyperosmolar non-ketotic coma (HONC) develops over days or weeks and is caused by inadequacy of insulin, resulting in severe hyperglycaemia
- In the UK, it accounts for approximately 2000 hospital admissions per year
- Mortality is high (15%), particularly in the elderly

Causes
- Infection is the most common cause
- Other causes include stressful events such as stroke, myocardial infarction, and surgery

Pathogenesis

The pathogenesis of HONC is similar to DKA, except that the patient does not develop ketoacidosis.

Investigations

As for DKA.

Diagnosis

- Blood glucose $>33.3\,mmol\,l^{-1}$
- pH >7.30
- Serum bicarbonate $>15\,mmol\,l^{-1}$
- Serum osmolality $>320\,mmol\,kg^{-1}$
- Trace of ketones in the urine

Treatment

As for DKA.

20 Management of hypoglycaemia

Definition:
- Hypoglycaemia is defined as a blood glucose level $< 4\,\text{mmol}\,\text{l}^{-1}$
- It is defined as 'mild' if self-treated and 'severe' if assistance by a third party is required

 Common misinterpretations and pitfalls

Hypoglycaemia can mimic any neurological presentation including coma, seizures, acute confusion, or isolated hemiparesis.

 NB Always exclude hypoglycaemia in any patient with coma.

Risks

- Altered consciousness can lead to airway compromise
- A prolonged severe hypoglycaemic episode can cause moderate to severe neuropsychological impairments
- Hypoglycaemia can cause an acute cerebral injury, causing hemiplegia

Incidence

- On average there are over 90 000 calls to the emergency services each year for hypoglycaemia in the UK
- In England, there are approximately 8000 admissions to hospital each year due to hypoglycaemia

Medical Student Survival Skills: The Acutely Ill Patient, First Edition. Philip Jevon, Konnur Ramkumar, and Emma Jenkinson.
© 2020 John Wiley & Sons Ltd. Published 2020 by John Wiley & Sons Ltd.
Companion website: www.wiley.com/go/jevon/medicalstudent

- At least 10% of in-patients in the UK have known diabetes. Being in hospital presents additional obstacles to maintaining good glycaemic control and avoiding hypoglycaemia. Hypoglycaemia occurs in 7.7% of admissions and prolongs hospital stay and increases mortality rates

Causes

- Too much insulin
- Delayed or missed meal or snack
- Not enough food, especially carbohydrates
- Unplanned or strenuous exercise
- Alcohol consumption without food
- Idiopathic

 Uncommon presentations

Occasionally hypoglycaemia can occur in a patient on sulphonylurea drugs – these patients must always be admitted and closely observed because there is a risk of hypoglycaemia reoccurring.

 NB Alcohol intake cause hypoglycaemia several hours later; the effects of alcohol may also mask hypoglycaemic symptoms.

Medical causes of hypoglycaemia include:

- Liver failure
- Addison's disease
- Pituitary insufficiency

Signs and symptoms

- These vary from person to person, although they are often constant for an individual
- They can be classified as either autonomic (usually present first when the blood glucose is 3.3–3.6 mmol l^{-1}), related to neuroglycopenia (usually present when the blood glucose is <2.6 mmol l^{-1}), or general malaise:
  - *Autonomic*: sweating, hunger, hot sensation, anxiety, nausea and vomiting

    – *Neuroglycopenia*: fatigue, visual disturbance, uncoordinated and altered behaviour, drowsiness, confusion, stroppy, moody, and if untreated convulsions and coma

    – *General malaise*: headache and nausea

(Edinburgh Hypoglycaemia Scale)

NB In patients with chronic hyperglycaemia, the autonomic clinical features may be triggered at higher blood glucose levels.

NB The patient is usually aware that he or she is developing hypoglycaemia, although this may not always be the case.
In addition, recurrent hypoglycaemic episodes can lead to diminished casualty awareness of impending hypoglycaemia.

Investigations

- Bedside blood glucose measurement should be undertaken

Diagnosis

- The biomedical diagnosis of hypoglycaemia is a blood sugar $<2.5\,\text{mmol}\,\text{l}^{-1}$

Treatment of hypoglycaemia

- ABCDE approach
- Treatment will depend upon the patient's conscious level and degree of cooperation
- If the patient's conscious level allows them to safely eat and drink, offer 15–20 g of fast-acting glucose, e.g. three to four glucose tablets or a glass of Lucozade. This can then be followed by long-acting carbohydrates, e.g. digestive biscuits. In some clinical settings, GlucoGel (formally known as Hypostop) (a dextrose gel, rapidly absorbed via the buccal mucosa) may be administered
- If the patient's conscious level has deteriorated, ensure their airway is clear and maintained; place patient in the lateral position. If the patient is unconscious, consider inserting a basic airway device, e.g. oropharyngeal airway

- Establish oxygen saturation monitoring using a pulse oximeter
- Administer high-flow oxygen using a non-rebreathe mask
- Insert a wide bore IV cannula (e.g. 14G)
- Administer 75–80 ml of 20% dextrose over 10–15 minutes
- If there is difficulty securing IV access, administer glucagon 1 mg IM
- Monitor blood glucose measurements
- Monitor the patient's response and conscious level; 90% of patients will fully recover in 20 minutes
- Try to establish the possible cause of the hypoglycaemia. To prevent a repeat hypoglycaemic episode, offer the patient food that contains starchy carbohydrates (absorbed more slowly), e.g. a sandwich, fruit, bowl of cereal, or biscuits and milk
- Educate the patient. Education is the key to preventing recurrent or severe hypoglycaemia. It may be necessary to involve the diabetes team
- Reassure the patient. Repeated episodes of hypoglycaemia may cause extreme emotional distress, even when the episodes are relatively mild

NB Remember the possible effects of concurrent use of drugs with hypoglycaemic agents, e.g. warfarin, quinine, salicylates, fibrates, sulphonamides, monoamine oxidase inhibitors, non-steroidal anti-inflammatory drugs, probenecid, somatostatin analogues, selected serotonin reuptake inhibitors.

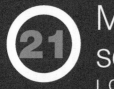

Management of severe headache

I. Chukwulobelu, G. S. Seyan, and G. R. Layton

Manor Hospital, Walsall, UK

> **Definitions:** Headache (or cephalgia) is defined as pain occurring above the orbitomeatal line.

Background

- The intensity of pain is usually expressed in terms of functional impact
- Sudden onset headaches take seconds to minutes to reach maximum intensity
- Headache affects an estimated 40% of people in the UK at some time in their lives and accounts for 1–2% of admissions to hospital

Classification

- Headache can be referred to as primary or secondary:
  - Primary headaches are not associated with organic disease or structural neurological abnormality
  - Secondary headaches are associated with demonstrable organic disease or attributable to a structural abnormality, confirmed by laboratory testing or imaging studies
- 90% of patients will have a primary (or idiopathic) headache syndrome but doctors should be sure to always perform a thorough assessment of every patient with headache in order to avoid missing a sinister secondary headache, which occur in 5–10% of cases.

Medical Student Survival Skills: The Acutely Ill Patient, First Edition. Philip Jevon, Konnur Ramkumar, and Emma Jenkinson.
© 2020 John Wiley & Sons Ltd. Published 2020 by John Wiley & Sons Ltd.
Companion website: www.wiley.com/go/jevon/medicalstudent

Primary headaches

- Migraine (without aura, with aura)
- Tension-type headache
- Cluster headache

Secondary headaches

- Vascular disease
- Infection (e.g. meningitis, encephalitis)
- Inflammation/immune-mediated (giant cell arteritis
- Space-occupying lesions
- Trauma
- Changes to intracranial pressure (Box 21.1)
- Metabolic, homeostatic, or toxic disturbances

Box 21.1 Features of raised intracranial pressure	
Headache	Typically worse when supine and in the morning
	Worsens with coughing and Valsalva activity
Vomiting	Vomiting without nausea in early stage
	Projectile vomiting with rising intracranial pressure
Ocular palsies	6th nerve palsy, 3rd nerve palsy
Altered consciousness	Decreasing Glasgow coma score (GCS), progressing to stupor and coma
Papilloedema	May cause optic atrophy if chronic
Cushing's triad	Increased systolic pressure with widened pulse pressure, bradycardia, and irregular breathing
	A late sign implying impending brain herniation

Clinical assessment of headache

History

- Take a detailed history in a systematic manner
- Use the SOCRATES (Box 21.2) approach in assessing pain, and be vigilant to qualify onset and red flag features
- Be sure to ask about occupational, sexual, travel, and immunisation history

Box 21.2 SOCRATES mnemonic for pain assessment	
S Site	T Time/duration
O Onset	E Exacerbating/relieving factors
C Character	S Severity (usually using a 0-10 pain scale)
R Radiation	
A Associated symptoms	

Red flags
- Sudden onset, reaching maximal intensity within <5 minutes
- Severity increasing over time (weeks to months) without remittance
- Worse in mornings
- Worse when coughing, bending, or going from sitting to standing (so-called postural association)
- Headache associated with focal neurological symptoms or signs
- Headaches associated with visual loss
- Past medical history or a current diagnosis of immunosuppression, cancer, or tuberculosis (Table 21.1)

ABCDE approach to examination and initial management

Table 21.1 ABCDE approach to the examination and initial management of headache

	Examine	Measure/monitor	Treat/intervention	Investigations
Airway	Assess for sounds of airway obstruction or compromise	O_2 saturations Capnography	Simple airway adjuncts if reduced GCS Contact anaesthetist if airway compromise (GCS <8)	
Breathing	Inspect, palpate, percuss, and auscultate	O2 saturations Respiratory rate	High-flow oxygen (15 l min^{-1}) via non-rebreathe mask(avoid hypercapnia as this can increase intracranial pressure)	Arterial blood gas (ABG) to assess for respiratory failure
Circulation	Inspect, palpate, and auscultate Assess for clinical evidence of carotid bruits or cardiovascular disease	Heart rate Blood pressure Assess for features of Cushing's triad (hypertension, bradycardia, altered respiratory pattern – late sign of raised intracranial pressure) Urine output Temperature	Secure IV access Consider bolus fluids if hypotensive – e.g. 500 ml crystalloid stat If hypertensive (blood pressure [BP] >180/110) discuss with senior Catheter	Bloods – FBC, U&Es, LFTs, Clotting, ABG/VBG Consider blood cultures Consider chest X-ray if signs of aspiration as a result of reduced GCS

(Continued)

Table 21.1 (Continued)

	Examine	Measure/monitor	Treat/intervention	Investigations
Disability	Perform a full cranial nerve examination Perform a full upper and lower neurological examination Check for signs of meningism – neck stiffness, Brudzinski's sign, Kernig's sign, photophobia Check for signs of raised intracranial pressure – fixed pupils, abnormal posturing, altered breathing Assess pupil size and response	Assess GCS Blood glucose (important for differentials)	Appropriate analgesia (see specific headaches) Blood glucose if <4 or >11 treat appropriately	Consider neuroimaging and lumbar puncture
Exposure	Assess for rashes Check temperature			Consider neuroimaging and lumbar puncture

NB Be aware!

If meningitis or encephalitis are suspected, delayed treatment can result in poor outcomes. Send samples (e.g. lumbar puncture) and start empirical treatment immediately without waiting for results of investigations.

Acute assessment and management of specific primary headaches

Migraine

'Common' migraine – with aura (~70%)

- Diagnosis requires:
  - History of five or more attacks
  - Four hours to 3 days in duration

- Two or more of the following:
  - Unilateral
  - Pulsating
  - Moderate or severe pain intensity
  - Worsened by or causing avoidance of routine physical activity
- One or more of the following:
  - Nausea and/or vomiting
  - Photophobia
  - Phonophobia

'Classic' migraine – without aura (~30%)

- Diagnosis is the same as above but also requires a history of two attacks that:
  - Have typical aura:
    - Visual, sensory, and/or speech symptoms that fully resolve
    - No motor symptoms
    - Visual symptoms – flashing lights (can be unilateral or bilateral), zig-zag lines, central scotoma, transient hemianopia
    - Sensory symptoms – typically unilateral paraesthesia
    - Speech symptoms – aphasia, dysarthria
    - Aura symptoms lasting between 5 and 60 minutes
  - Aura is typically preceded, accompanied, or followed by headache within 60 minutes (~40% experience aura without headache)
  - Atypical aura – associated with motor features
- It is not possible to diagnose a first headache as migraine without ruling out other differentials
- Be cautious in diagnosing a migraine if the headache or aura is atypical for the patient or there is residual neurology post-headache
- Assess and stabilise patient using the ABCDE approach
- Nurse the patient in a darkened room

Management of common and classic migraine

- Combination therapy, first line: offer oral triptan (sumatriptan 50–100 mg PO or sumatriptan 6 mg SC) and non-steroidal anti-inflammatory drug (NSAID) (ibuprofen 600 mg PO), or oral triptan and paracetamol
- If monotherapy is preferred: offer oral triptan, NSAID, or aspirin (900 mg PO) in isolation
- Add in antiemetic: dopamine antagonist, e.g. metoclopramide (10 mg IV)
- Discharge with GP follow-up, and explain the importance of trigger avoidance and basis of self-management
- Avoid using ergot-based derivatives for the management of migraine

> **NB** Be aware!
> All triptans are contraindicated in patients with known coronary artery disease, previous myocardial infarction, or possible undiagnosed coronary artery disease.

Cluster headache

- Rapid onset of very severe 'stabbing' pain around/behind one eye
- Associated with red, watery eye, miosis, ptosis, and nasal congestion – patients describe pacing around the room
- Attacks last between 15 and 180 minutes, occurring once or twice per day, and are typically nocturnal
- Attacks occur in clusters lasting between 4 and 12 weeks with periods of remission lasting 3 months to 3 years
- More common in men
- Triggered by alcohol and smoking

Management

- Sumatriptan 6 mg SC provided there are no contraindications
- Short burst oxygen therapy: 100% oxygen at 12–15 l min^{-1} for 15–20 minutes
- Verapamil may be used for prophylaxis
- Avoid paracetamol, NSAIDs, opioids, ergots, and oral triptans
- Discharge patient to GP, and discuss trigger avoidance and basis of self-management

Tension headache

- This is the most common form of headache
- It is a chronic 'tight band'-like headache with generalised constant pain, often described as a 'dull ache', frequently worse in the evenings, and there may be tenderness
- The most common triggers are stress and musculoskeletal problems
- More common in females
- There is no photophobia, neck stiffness, or vomiting and no neurology

Management

- Reassure the patient
- Conservative measures include management of stress, mood disorders, and sleep disorders

- Use paracetamol and NSAIDs, and avoid the use of opioids
- Low dose amitriptyline or acupuncture can be used for prophylaxis

Acute assessment and management of secondary headaches

Subarachnoid haemorrhage

Subarachnoid haemorrhage (SAH) involves bleeding of vessels that lie in the subarachnoid space, the area between the arachnoid membrane and pia mater. Most occur as a result of the rupture of an intracranial aneurysm (~80%), whilst others may occur as a result of arterial venous malformations (~10%).

Risk factors
- Smoking
- Hypertension
- Alcohol
- Family history (3–5× increased risk)
- Female (above the age of 50 years)
- Bleeding disorders

Berry aneurysm association
- Autosomal dominant polycystic kidney disease
- Ehlers–Danlos syndrome
- Coarctation of aorta

Signs and symptoms
- Sudden, severe, 'thunderclap' occipital headache
  - 30–50% experience 'sentinel headaches' – warning headaches as a result of smaller bleeds or aneurysmal expansion
- Meningism (neck stiffness, photophobia, Kernig's sign)
- Reduced GCS (drowsiness, coma)
- Seizure

Complications
- Rebleeding
- Cerebral ischaemia
- Obstructive hydrocephalus

Specific investigations
- Coagulation screen
- Non-contrast computed tomography scan of the head (99% sensitive in the first 6 hours)
- Lumbar puncture (12 hours after onset of headache)
  - Specifically to look for xanthochromia (sample should be shielded from light)

Management
- Bed rest
- Nimodipine (60 mg PO 4 hourly for 21 days) to prevent cerebral vasospasm
- Neurosurgical referral (coiling > clipping)

Giant cell arteritis

A large vessel vasculitis associated with an inflamed and tender temporal artery.

Risk factors
- Female (1% lifetime risk)
- Advanced aged (peak between 70 and 79 years, almost never before 50)
- Scandinavian descent
- Past medical history of polymyalgia rheumatica

Signs and symptoms
- Unilateral headache
- Systemic features (fever, malaise, anorexia, weight loss)
- Scalp tenderness
- Jaw claudication
- Visual loss (red flag)

Complications
- Anterior ischaemic optic neuropathy
- Central retinal artery occlusion
- Aortic vasculitis pathology (aneurysm, dissection)

Specific investigations
- Full blood count (raised erythrocyte sedimentation rate)
- Temporal artery biopsy (may produce false negatives due to skip lesions)

Specific management

- High dose steroid (e.g. prednisolone 40–60 mg PO)
- If there are any visual symptoms seek an urgent ophthalmology review
- Proton pump inhibitor cover for high dose steroids

Hypertensive emergency/hypertensive encephalopathy

A hypertensive emergency is defined as severe hypertension (BP >180/110) with acute end organ damage. Hypertensive encephalopathy is characterised by severe hypertension (BP >180/110) associated with headache, confusion, and papilloedema.

Risk factors

- Non-compliance with antihypertensive medications
- Renovascular disease
- Autoimmune disease
- Recreational drug use (cocaine, amphetamines)
- Pregnancy

Signs and symptoms

- Seizures
- Decreased GCS
- Retinal haemorrhages
- Blurring of vision
- Nausea and/or vomiting

Specific investigations

- Fundoscopy – assess for grade IV retinal features of hypertensive retinopathy – papilloedema, haemorrhage, exudates, and cotton wool spots
- ECG

Specific management

- Hypertensive encephalopathy should be managed in an intensive treatment unit setting with IV antihypertensives, where this is not available oral alternatives can be used
- IV labetalol can be given as a 20 mg bolus followed by further 20–80 mg boluses every 10 minutes (maximum dose 300 mg) *or* it can be given as a continuous infusion of 0.5–2 mg min^{-1}
- Oral alternatives include single dose nifedipine 10 mg or sublingual captopril 25 mg

- Aim to reduce the mean arterial blood pressure (MAP) by 10–20% within the first hour; further treatment should not lower the MAP by more than 25% in the first 24 hours

> **NB** Be aware!
> Be cautious when reducing blood pressure in hypertensive emergencies, as rapid lowering could lead to ischaemic strokes in watershed areas of arterial supply.

Acute angle closure glaucoma

Acute angle closure can lead to glaucoma – suspect acute angle closure in the following circumstances:
- Acutely red, painful eye with blurred vision and/or headaches
- Associated with nausea and seeing halos around lights due to hazy cornea
- The pupil is semidilated and fixed, it may be oval-shaped
- On gentle palpation, the eye may feel tender and hard, with raised intraocular pressure on tonometry
- Symptoms typically occur in the evening and are worse in low light
- Precipitating factors for acute angle closure include prolonged pupillary dilation, e.g. watching television in a darkened room, adrenergic drugs (e.g. phenylephrine) or antimuscarinic drugs (e.g. tricyclic antidepressants)
- More common in middle aged, elderly, and hypermetropic (long-sighted) individuals

Management
- Admit for specialist assessment and treatment by ophthalmologist
- Keep in well-lit environment and avoid anything that causes pupil dilation
- Lie flat on back with face up to reduce angle pressure (do not support the head with pillows)
- Use topical pilocarpine drops – one drop of 2% in blue eyes, one drop of 4% in brown eyes
- Acetazolamide 500 mg PO (reduces production of aqueous humour)
- Analgesia – e.g. morphine 2.5 mg IV for severe pain
- Antiemetic – e.g. metoclopramide 10 mg IV

22 Management of acute liver failure

N Gautam

Manor Hospital, Walsall, UK

Definition: Acute liver failure (ALF) is a rare condition in which rapid deterioration of liver function results in an altered mental state (encephalopathy) and coagulopathy (international normalised ratio [INR] > 1.5) in a previously healthy individual.

NB Acute liver failure carries a very high mortality in young individuals.

Classification

The classification of ALF is based on the duration of time between the development of jaundice to the onset of encephalopathy (Table 22.1).

Table 22.1 Classification of ALF (time from jaundice to onset of encephalopathy)

Definition	Time (days)	Most common aetiologies	Definition (weeks)	Time
Hyperacute	< 7 days	Paracetamol (acetominophen) overdose (POD), hepatitis A and B	Fulminant	< 2 weeks
Acute	8–28 days	POD, hepatitis A, B, and E		
Subacute	29 days–8 weeks	Idiosyncratic drug reactions, seronegative hepatitis	Subfulminant	> 2 weeks

Incidence

- There are approximately 400 cases in the UK annually
- 70% of cases are secondary to paracetamol use

Medical Student Survival Skills: The Acutely Ill Patient, First Edition. Philip Jevon, Konnur Ramkumar, and Emma Jenkinson.
© 2020 John Wiley & Sons Ltd. Published 2020 by John Wiley & Sons Ltd.
Companion website: www.wiley.com/go/jevon/medicalstudent

- There are 1–6 cases/year/million population in the developing world.
- Viral hepatitis (hepatitis B) is the leading cause of ALF in the developing world (Table 22.2)

Table 22.2 Common causes of ALF

Drug-induced	Viral causes	Other causes
Acetaminophen (N-acetyl-p-aminophenol)	Hepatitis A, B, C, E	Acute fatty liver of pregnancy
Isoniazid	Cytomegalovirus	Lymphoma
Propylthiouracil	Epstein–Barr virus	Ischemic hepatitis
Phenytoin	Herpes simplex virus	Acute Budd–Chiari syndrome
Valproate		Acute Wilson's disease
		Autoimmune disease
		Peripartum cardiomyopathy

Clinical features

- *Whole body*
  - Systemic inflammatory response
  - High energy expenditure and catabolism
- *Liver*
  - Loss of metabolic function
  - Decreased gluconeogenesis leading to hypoglycaemia
  - Decreased lactate clearance leading to lactic acidosis
  - Decreased ammonia clearance leading to hyperammonaemia
  - Decreased synthetic capacity leading to coagulopathy
- *Lungs*
  - Acute lung injury
  - Adult respiratory distress syndrome
- *Adrenal gland*
  - Inadequate glucocorticoid production contributing to hypotension
- *Bone marrow*
  - Frequent suppression, especially in viral and seronegative disease
- *Circulating leucocytes*
  - Impaired function and immunoparesis contributing to high risk of sepsis
- *Brain*
  - Hepatic encephalopathy
  - Cerebral oedema
  - Intracranial hypertension

- *Heart*
  - High output state
  - Frequent subclinical myocardial injury
- *Pancreatitis*
  - Particularly in paracetamol-related ALF
- *Kidney*
  - Frequent dysfunction or failure
- *Portal hypertension*
  - Might be prominent in subacute disease and confused with chronic liver disease

(Source: Bernal et al. 2010)

History taking

In taking the history, focus on the following:
- Date of onset of jaundice and encephalopathy
- Alcohol use
- Medication use (prescription, illicit, and recreational)
- Herbal or traditional medicine use
- Family history of liver disease (Wilson's disease)
- Exposure risk factors for viral hepatis (travel, transfusions, sexual contacts, occupation, tattoos)
- Exposure to hepatic toxins (mushrooms, organic solvents)
- Evidence of complications (e.g. renal failure, seizures, bleeding, infection)
- Psychiatric history

Investigations

Bloods
- Full bloods count – look for thrombocytopenia
- Renal function – renal failure is common
- INR or prothrombin time (PT) – prolonged
- Arterial blood gases (ABGs) – metabolic acidosis, hypoxemia
- Lactate – high lactate
- Liver function tests (LFTs) – may have high bilirubin, Marked transaminitis in PCM poisoning
- Phosphate – high phosphate marker of impaired liver regeneration
- Blood glucose – may be dangerously low

- Ammonia – high ammonia is suggestive of cerebral oedema
- Blood culture – sepsis

Diagnostic tests

The diagnostic tests that should be requested depend on the clinical situation.

- Viral screen (immunoglobulin M [IgM] hepatitis A virus, IgM anti-HBc, hepatitis C and E virus)
- Copper, caeruloplasmin
- Autoantibodies (include anti-liver-kidney microsomal antibody)
- Immunoglobulins
- Pregnancy test (where appropriate)
- Clotting studies
- Ultrasound looking at hepatic vasculature
- Computed tomography scan

Initial management

- ABCDE approach
- Ensure safe environment for patient (may be confused)
- Attach monitoring – blood pressure, pulse oximetry, and electrocardiogram
- Target oxygen therapy
- Involve senior help early
- Avoid all sedating agents unless intubated, non-steroidal anti-inflammatory drugs, and any IM injection
- Administer vitamin K 10 mg IV once daily in 1–2 doses
- Aggressive fluid resuscitation
- Maintain strict fluid balance chart; daily weights may be helpful
- Administer broad-spectrum IV antibiotics/antifungals, e.g. tazocin
- Administer IV proton pump inhibitor, e.g. ranitidine 50 mg twice a day to prevent stress ulcers
- Monitor blood glucose
- Request nutritional support: advice from the dietician
- Early involvement of nearest liver centre (Table 22.3)
- Liver transplant is the definitive treatment for ALF (Table 22.4)

Table 22.3 Criteria for discussion with and transfer to nearest specialist liver centre

| Organ system | Paracetamol overdose (time from ingestion, days) | | | Non-paracetamol overdose (ALF classification, time from jaundice to encephalopathy) | | |
	Day 2	Day 3	Day 4	Hyperacute	Acute	Subacute
Liver	INR >3.0 or PT >50s	INR >4.5 or PT >75s	INR >6 or PT >100s	INR >2.0 or PT >30s	INR >2.0 or PT >30s	INR >1.5 or PT >20s or shrinking liver volume
Metabolic	pH <7.3 or HCO$_3$ <16 or lactate >3.0 or hypoglycaemia	pH <7.3 or HCO$_3$ <16 or lactate >3.0		Hypoglycaemia or hyperpyrexia	Hypoglycaemia	Hypoglycaemia or hyponatraemia <130 umol l^{-1}
Kidney	Oliguria or serum creatinine (SCr) >200 umol l^{-1}	Oliguria or SCr >200 umol l^{-1}	Oliguria or SCr >300 umol l^{-1}	Acute kidney injury (AKI)	AKI	AKI
Brain	Hepatic encephalopathy (HE)	HE	HE	HE	HE	HE
Haematology		Severe thromabocytopenia	Severe thromabocytopenia			

Source: Slack and Wendon (2011).

Table 22.4 Kings College criteria for super urgent listing for orthotopic liver transplantation

Organ system	Paracetamol overdose	Seronegative hepatitis (SNH), hepatitis A, hepatitis B, or an idiosyncratic drug reaction (IDR)
Liver	*MUST* occur within 24 hour time window	INR >6.5 or PT >100 s
	INR >6.5 or PT >100 s with both	with any grade of HE
	AKI stage 3 and grade 3/4 HE	and three of the following: INR >3.5 or PT >50 s; bilirubin >300 umol l⁻¹; jaundice to HE >7 days; unfavourable aetiology SNH or IDR; age >40 years
Metabolic	pH <7.25 or lactate >3.0 mmol l⁻¹ (after >24 hours after overdose despite aggressive fluid resuscitation usually in addition to O'Grady criteria to increase sensitivity and specificity)	
Kidney	AKI stage 3 (SCr >300 umol l⁻¹ or anuria) with both INR >6.5 or PT >100 s *and* grade 3/4 HE	
Brain	Grade 3/4 HE with both INR >6.5 or PT >100 s *and* AKI stage 3	Any grade of HE with INR >6.5 or PT >100 s
Cardiac	In the UK, increased inotrope or vasopressor requirement in the absence of sepsis with 2 out of 3: INR >6.5 or PT >100 s; AK stage 3; grade 3/4 HE	

Source: Slack and Wendon (2011).

> **NB** *N*-acetylcysteine is used in paracetamol poisoning:
> - Should be given in 5% glucose by IV infusion
> - Loading dose: 150 mg kg⁻¹ in 200 ml over 15 minutes
> - Followed by 50 mg kg⁻¹ in 500 ml over 4 hours
> - Followed by maintenance regime: dose 100 mg kg⁻¹ body weight, diluted in 1000 ml 5% dextrose, given at 62.5 ml h⁻¹

Summary

OSCE Key Learning Points

✔ Life-threatening condition that can lead to multiorgan failure and death
✔ History is crucial
✔ Early recognition and treatment is key
✔ Ensure early involvement of nearest specialist liver unit

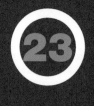

23 Management of self-harm and poisoning

I. Chukwulobelu and G. S. Seyan

Manor Hospital, Walsall, UK

Definition:
- Deliberate self-harm is an acute, non-fatal act carried out to cause harm
- Poisoning is taking a substance that causes health hazards. This can be done accidentally or deliberately, with the intention of self-harm or suicide

Incidence

- Deliberate self-harm has an annual incidence of 2–3/1000 people (rates are likely to be underestimated)
- Deliberate self-harm accounts for ~10% of all acute medical admissions in the UK
- Deliberate self-harm is more common in young females, with a worrying increase in incidence of 68% amongst girls aged 13–16 years since 2011
- Conversely, successful suicide attempts are more common in young males
- Self-poisoning accounts for 90% of medical presentations of deliberate self-harm
- Overdoses account for ~15% of acute medical emergencies
- Risk factors are listed in Box 23.1

Medical Student Survival Skills: The Acutely Ill Patient, First Edition. Philip Jevon, Konnur Ramkumar, and Emma Jenkinson.
© 2020 John Wiley & Sons Ltd. Published 2020 by John Wiley & Sons Ltd.
Companion website: www.wiley.com/go/jevon/medicalstudent

Box 23.1 Risk factors

Deliberate self-harm	Risk factors for suicide
Female	Male
History of mental health disease (personality disorders, autism)	History of mental health disease (especially depression and schizophrenia)
Triggering life events (e.g. abuse, unemployment, prison)	Prior suicide attempts (strongest predictive factor)
Lesbian, gay, bisexual, transgender, questioning (LGBTQ) population	Elderly population
Younger population	Chronic medical conditions (terminal and painful diseases)

Common risk factors

Low socioeconomic status
Alcohol abuse
Social isolation

Assessment and diagnosis of patients presenting with self-harm

History

- Ascertaining an accurate history may be difficult for the following reasons:
  - Reduced Glasgow coma score (GCS) as a result of poison
  - Altered mental state and psychosis as a result of poison
  - Inaccurate information as a result of an underlying mental health disorder
- Collateral history often provides invaluable information for discerning what drugs may have been taken and the circumstances around the overdose
- It is important to identify those with *genuine suicidal ideation* and those with risk of future self-harm. Features that indicate a genuine attempt are as follows:
  - Premeditation (preparation of a will, suicide notes, financial preparation)
  - Expected fatal outcome
  - Associated drug and alcohol use
  - Violent methods used
  - Precautions to discovery
  - Regret at failed attempt
- Suicide risk assessment tools are widely used in NHS trusts but have little evidence of being able to appropriately stratify patient risk; approximately 1% of patients presenting with self-harm will go on to commit suicide

- Overall clinical impression and intuition should not be ignored in the assessment of patients presenting with self-harm (Table 23.1)

 NB Be aware!
Asking about suicidal ideation does not increase risk of suicide.

- Emergency treatment of poisoning should be according to Toxbase www.toxbase.org (username and password are available at each trust – if you do not know, ask in the emergency department)
- Toxbase is an invaluable resource that will provide detailed information on the toxins present in any formulae
- If any further information is required, contact your local poisons service or call the UK National Poisons Information Service on 0844 8920111

ABCDE approach to examination and management

Table 23.1 ABCDE approach to the examination and initial management of self-harm and poisoning

	Examine	Measure/monitor	Treat/intervention	Investigations
Airway	Assess for sounds of airway obstruction or compromise	O_2 saturations Capnography	Simple airway adjuncts if reduced GCS Contact anaesthetist if airway compromise (GCS <8)	
Breathing	Inspect, palpate, percuss, and auscultate Assess for any signs of aspiration	O_2 saturations – may appear cyanosed or flushed Respiratory rate – may have respiratory depression or tachypnoea If respiratory depression, consider naloxone 400 µg	High-flow oxygen (15 l min^{-1}) via non-rebreathe mask	Arterial blood gas (ABG) to assess for respiratory failure and metabolic acidosis (e.g. paracetamol, aspirin, and tricyclic antidepressant poisoning)

(Continued)

Table 23.1 (Continued)

	Examine	Measure/monitor	Treat/intervention	Investigations
Circulation	Inspect, palpate, and auscultate Check capillary refill and jugular venous pressure	Heart rate – may have tachycardia or bradycardia Blood pressure – may be hypotensive Urine output	Secure IV access – two wide bore cannulas Consider bolus fluids if hypotensive – e.g. 500 ml crystalloid stat Catheterise and monitor urine output – aim at 0.5 ml kg^{-1} h^{-1}	Bloods – full blood count, urea and electrolytes (U&Es), liver function tests (LFTs), clotting, ABG/venous blood gas Drug levels (paracetamol and salicylate) Electrocardiogram (ECG) – to look for specific pathology (e.g. broadening QRS in tricyclic depression overdose, ST elevation in cocaine use) Consider blood cultures Consider chest X-ray if signs of aspiration
Disability	Assess pupil size and response If reduced GCS then perform a full cranial nerve examination, and upper and lower limb neurological examination	Assess GCS Blood glucose (important for differentials)	Appropriate analgesia Blood glucose if <4 or >11 treat appropriately	Consider neuroimaging
Exposure	Assess for signs of IV drug use Check temperature Digital rectal examination or per vaginal examination to assess if patient has concealed drugs		Consider detaining patient under Mental Health Act if appropriate	Obtain collateral history Check Toxbase for specific management of poisoning

Poisoning

Principles of poisons management are as follows:

- Resuscitation of the patient
- Reducing the absorption of the poison if possible
- Giving specific antidotes if available (Table 23.2)

Table 23.2 Drug antidotes

Drug	Antidote
Beta-blockers	Glucagon, atropine
Benzodiazepines	Flumazenil if severe (use with caution)
Digoxin	Digibind
Ethylene glycerol	Fomepizole (better than ethanol)
Iron tablet	Desferrioxamine
Opiates	Naloxone

Common poisons include:
- Paracetamol
- Opiates
- Benzodiazepines
- Alcohol
- Antidepressants
- Aspirin

NB Be aware!
- 50% of patients will have also consumed alcohol
- 30% of patients will have taken multiple drugs

Signs and symptoms

Sign	Potential drug
Hypoventilation	Opiates, ethanol, benzodiazepines
Hyperventilation	Salicylic acid, carbon monoxide
Miosis	Opiates, acetylcholinergics
Dilated pupils	Anticholinergics
Bradycardia	Beta-blockers, digoxin
Tachyarrhythmias	Tricyclic antidepressants, lithium, cocaine
Hyperthermia	Ecstasy, amphetamines, SSRIs

Specific poisons

Paracetamol

In overdose, treatment is focused on restoring stores of glutathione to remove the toxic metabolite of paracetamol, N-acetyl-p-benzoquinone (NABQI).

- < 24 hours: overdose symptoms are often mild and potentially asymptomatic
- 24–36 hours: right upper quadrant pain may have developed due to hepatic necrosis with associated signs of acute liver failure (jaundice, encephalopathy)
- Encephalopathy can worsen over the next 72 hours

Specific management

If the time of overdose is known then ideally blood levels should be taken at four hours post ingestion: once the levels are known then the following nomogram (Figure 23.1) is used to determine whether or not treatment should be commenced. Acetylcysteine should be commenced within eight hours of ingestion, therefore if there is any anticipated delay in obtaining blood levels before this time then treatment should be commenced whilst levels are pending.

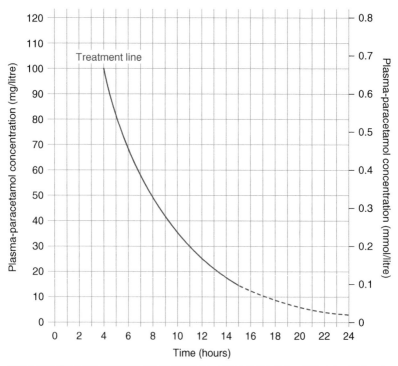

Figure 23.1 Treatment nomogram for paracetamol overdose (British National Formulary/Toxbase).

The following treatment regime should be used:

- First infusion: acetylcysteine 150 mg kg^{-1} in 200 ml 5% dextrose over 1 hour
- Second infusion: acetylcysteine 50 mg kg^{-1} in 500 ml 5% dextrose over 4 hours
- Third infusion: acetylcysteine 100 mg kg^{-1} in 1000 ml % dextrose over 16 hours. The 16 hourly infusion should continue until LFTs have been rechecked (seek senior advice)

NB Be aware!
In staggered paracetamol overdose (i.e. where tablets have been taken over a period of greater than one hour), blood levels are not useful for guiding the need for treatment, therefore acetylcysteine should be started immediately.

Liver transplantation

Indications for liver transplantation are according the King's College criteria (see Table 22.4):

- Arterial pH < 7.3, 24 hours after ingestion
- Or all of the following:
  - Prothrombin time (PT) > 100 seconds
  - Creatinine > 300 µmol l^{-1}
  - Grade III or IV encephalopathy

NB Be aware!
Remember patient trends and blood test trends are also important. Refer early if worsening PT, creatinine, or encephalopathy to allow the liver unit to assess and plan for a new patient.

Opiates

Overdosing usually occurs as a result of recreational use, but be wary of overdosing in patients who are opiate naïve or had dosing increased as part of chronic pain management.

Signs may include

- Respiratory depression is the cardinal feature of opioid toxicity (respiratory rate < 12)

- Pinpoint pupils (absence does not exclude possibility of toxicity)
- Reduced GCS
- Constipation

Specific management
- Initiate respiratory support using a bag–valve–mask if there are signs of severe respiratory depression (respiratory rate <8) and/or type respiratory failure on ABG
- Administer 400 μg of naloxone IV
  - IM and intranasal administration can be considered where IV access is not available, but they have unpredictable distribution profiles
  - The half-life of naloxone is shorter than opiates, so regular review is required
  - Giving enough naloxone to completely reverse the effects of opiates is *not* recommended. This can precipitate withdrawal symptoms and reverse pain control

NB Be aware!
Methadone and loperamide can cause prolonged QTc.

Aspirin (salicylic acid)

This is one of the most common drugs used in deliberate overdose. Moderate overdose patients present with the following:
- Tinnitus
- Epigastric pain
- Sweating
- Vomiting
- Blurring of vision

In adults a respiratory alkalosis initially develops as salicylic acid stimulates the central respiratory centres. A metabolic acidosis with a raised anion gap develops afterwards.

NB Be aware!
- Children are at risk of Reye's syndrome from taking aspirin – a condition that leads to encephalopathy and liver damage
- Children tend to only present with metabolic acidosis in aspirin overdose

Specific management

- Gastric lavage can be attempted within an hour of ingestion following large overdoses
- Urinary alkalinisation with sodium bicarbonate helps with elimination of aspirin, e.g. 1 L 1.26% $NaHCO_3$ with close monitoring of potassium
- Haemodialysis is indicated where there are the following:
  - Serum salicylate concentration $>700\,mg\,l^{-1}$
  - Metabolic acidosis refractory to treatment
  - Acute renal failure
  - Pulmonary oedema
  - Seizures
  - Coma

Tricyclic antidepressants

- Tricyclic antidepressants (TCAs) are highly toxic in overdose and can be fatal in doses 10× the daily dose
- Medications are lipophilic and protein bound so *cannot be dialysed*
- First generation TCAs are more likely to cause lethal intoxication
- Early signs are often related to the anticholinergic effects of TCAs:
  - Dry mouth
  - Dilated pupils
  - Tachycardia
  - Urinary retention

Specific management

- Patients with a reduced GCS should be managed in an intensive treatment unit (ITU) or high dependency unit (HDU) setting
- Gastric lavage and activated charcoal (50 g orally) should be given if the patient is seen with 1 hour of ingestion
- Ensure that an ECG is done on patients with suspected TCA poisoning
- Boluses of 50 mmol of 8.4% sodium bicarbonate IV should be given if there are either of the following:
  - Prolonged QRS duration
  - Metabolic acidosis

Selective serotonin reuptake inhibitors

- Common examples include fluoxetine, citalopram, and sertraline
- They are typically well tolerated in overdoses

- Ingestion of 30× the normal dose typically presents with minor or no symptoms at all. Ingestion of 50–75× the normal dose may cause vomiting and mild central nervous system depression
- Problems mainly arise when two serotonergics are ingested together, which may lead to 'serotonin syndrome'

Signs of serotonin syndrome
- Altered mental state
- Pyrexia
- Hyperreflexia
- Rigidity
- Dilated pupils
- Increased creatine kinase

Management of serotonin syndrome
- IV fluids
- Benzodiazepines
- In severe cases, give cyproheptadine

Cocaine

Cocaine is typically snorted or smoked (freebasing). This drug can present as massive overdosing when concealed packets (i.e. swallowed or per rectum) rupture; 1 g of pure cocaine is lethal.

Signs and symptoms
- Hypertension
- Pyrexia
- Agitation
- Seizures
- Tachycardia
- Chest pain

Complications
- Rhabdomyolysis
- Renal failure
- Psychosis
- Cerebrovascular events
- Myocardial infarction (related to vasospasm)

Specific management
- Give benzodiazepines to settle agitation
- Perform an ECG to look for any ischaemia and treat as an acute coronary syndrome or arrhythmias and treat according Resuscitation Council (UK) guidelines

Synthetic cannabinoids

These are a group of heterogeneous compounds that are designed to stimulate cannabinoid receptors. These compounds can range from two to 800 times more potent that their natural occurring counterparts. Initially designed to bypass drug legislation (now illegal), these drugs have seen a worrying increase of use in the twenty-first century.

Commonly known in the UK as Black Mamba its use is particularly prevalent amongst the homeless and prison populations. Given the variable nature of the compounds present, these drugs have the potential to cause serious and life-threatening toxicity.

Presentations of severe toxicity
- Florid toxic psychosis – similar to schizophrenia
- Coma
- Seizure
- Rhadomylosis
- Hyperthermia
- Respiratory arrest

Management
- Management is largely supportive
- ITU admission is common

Cardiopulmonary arrest

- Perform standard advanced life support (ALS)
- Give antidote/reversal agent if appropriate
- Consider magnesium sulphate if polymorphic VT (torsades de pointes) is the cause of the arrest

Prior to discharge

- Crisis team/psychiatric team input (check local policy)

OSCE Key Learning Points

✔ Consider poisoning in any unconscious adult with unknown cause
✔ Call for senior help early (SBAR)
✔ Refer to Toxbase for the specific management of poisons
✔ Staggered paracetamol overdose, start treatment without waiting for levels

Background

- Trauma is the commonest cause of loss of life in those aged under 44 years
- Estimated to be second commonest cause of 'life years lost' to death/disability worldwide by 2020
- 10 000 people in England/Wales die from trauma each year
- The commonest cause of trauma in the UK is from road traffic collisions

Pathophysiology

- Depends on mechanism of injury (Box 24.1)
- It may involve systemic injury and/or specific organ injury
- *Immediate death* may occur due to asphyxia or exsanguination
- *Early deaths* occur due to failure to manage ABCDE problems
- *Late deaths* occur due to complications

Box 24.1 Types of trauma

- *Blunt trauma*: e.g. pedestrian hit by car, hit by baseball bat
- *Penetrating trauma*: e.g. gunshot wound, stabbing
- *Environmental trauma*: e.g. electrocution, burns, frostbite

Pre-hospital management and handover

- Most patients with significant trauma arrive by ambulance
- Ambulance staff should hand over using ATMIST (Box 24.2)
- Initial assessment/resuscitation will usually have begun pre-hospital

Medical Student Survival Skills: The Acutely Ill Patient, First Edition. Philip Jevon,
Konnur Ramkumar, and Emma Jenkinson.
© 2020 John Wiley & Sons Ltd. Published 2020 by John Wiley & Sons Ltd.
Companion website: www.wiley.com/go/jevon/medicalstudent

Box 24.2 ATMIST handover	
A	Age/sex of patient
T	Time of incident
M	Mechanism of injury
I	Injuries (found *or* suspected)
S	Signs – vital signs *and* trends (improving *or* deteriorating)
T	Treatment – what treatment has already been initiated?

Assessment

- The *primary survey* involves the assessment/treatment of immediately life-threatening problems using ABCDE
- The *secondary survey* is only commenced once the patient is stable – it involves a full head to toe assessment of the patient, aiming to detecting *all* injuries, however minor

Primary survey

- ABCDE approach (Box 24.3)
- Treat problems as you find them
- Reassessment is key

Box 24.3 Primary survey	
A	Airway (with cervical spine control)
B	Breathing
C	Circulation
D	Disability
E	Environment/Exposure

Airway (with cervical spine control)

Assess the airway for:

- Visible obstructions (e.g. swelling, blood, foreign bodies)
- Noise (e.g. gurgling, stridor)
- *Potential* obstructions (e.g. singed hairs, carbon deposits, reduced conscious level)

Interventions

- Manual manoeuvres (e.g. chin lift, jaw thrust, *not* head tilt)
- Adjuncts (e.g. naso- or oropharyngeal airways)

NB

- The use of a nasopharyngeal airway is contraindicated in a potential base of skull fracture (i.e. patients with obvious head/facial injury)
- An oropharyngeal airway is unlikely to be tolerated in any patient not deeply unconscious (i.e. AVPU ≤P (see Box 24.11), Glasgow coma score ≤8)

- Administer oxygen 15 l min⁻¹ via a non-rebreathe oxygen mask
- Definitive airway, e.g. ETT or surgical airway, is likely to require a specialist: call for help early

Manage the *cervical spine* with:

- Manual in-line immobilisation
- Consider triple immobilisation (with correctly fitting collar, blocks and tape) in patients where there is any doubt about the patient's ability to protect their own cervical spine, however exercise caution in patients with significant head injuries, where a tightly-fitting collar can worsen intracranial hypertension.

Breathing

Assess breathing (look, listen, feel) for:

- External signs of injury (wounds, bruising, deformity, tracheal deviation)
- Excursion (accessory muscle use, paradoxical movements)
- Decreased/absent air entry
- Tenderness/crepitus

Breathing problems that must be addressed

- Tension pneumothorax (Box 24.4) (needle thoracocentesis – Box 24.5)
- Open pneumothorax (three-way occlusive dressing – Box 24.6)

Box 24.4 Signs of tension pneumothorax

- Severe respiratory distress
- Pain
- Absence of breath sounds on affected side
- Hyperresonance on affected side
- Tachycardia
- Hypotension
- Tracheal deviation away from side of injury

Box 24.5 Needle thoracocentesis

- Landmark: 2nd intercostal space, mid-clavicular line (on affected side)
- Equipment: antiseptic swab, large bore needle
- Aiming to release the tension, i.e. convert to simple pneumothorax
- Must follow up with a chest drain as soon as possible

Box 24.6 Treatment of open pneumothorax

- Apply a non-adherent dressing and occlude it on *three* sides, not four

- Massive haemothorax (IV access and early chest drain – Box 24.7)
- Flail chest/pulmonary contusion (analgesia/early intubation)
- Cardiac tamponade (pericardiocentesis/early surgery)

Box 24.7 Treatment of massive haemothorax

- Get good intravenous access first
- Use open technique for chest drain insertion
- Use 'triangle of safety' (4–5th intercostal space, latissimus dorsi posteriorly, pectoralis major anteriorly, aiming anterior to mid-axillary line
- Ensure full personal protective equipment/sterile techniques
- Provide adequate analgesia/anaesthesia
- Make large skin incision insertion (immediately above rib, avoiding neurovascular bundle)
- Blunt dissect using artery forceps until through the pleura
- Finger-sweep to ensure there is no palpable liver, etc.
- Insert large drain using instrument, ensuring all holes are inside the chest
- Suture the drain securely
- Apply dressing to prevent accidental dislodging but allowing full view of incision site
- If patient drains > 1 l of blood discuss with thoracic surgeons as soon as possible

Circulation

Assess circulation (look, listen, feel) for:
- Heart sounds
- Pulse (volume/rate)
- Blood pressure
- Capillary refill time
- Signs of bleeding (chest, abdomen, pelvis, long bones, external bleeding)

Interventions
- Direct compression on bleeding wounds
- Compression on proximal arteries if above is not successful
- Application of tourniquet if above fails
- Adequate circulatory access (Box 24.8)
- Consideration of fluid requirement (e.g. 2 l crystalloid early if patient is shocked)
- Early consideration of blood (Box 24.9 – consider massive transfusion)

Box 24.8 Options for immediate access in trauma patients

- Intravenous (anterior cubital fossa or external jugular, hand or foot)
- Intraosseous (proximal tibial, distal femoral, proximal humerus)
- Central (subclavian, femoral, internal jugular)
- Venous cut-down (long saphenous vein)

Box 24.9 Options for blood requesting

- O-negative (immediately available if required)
- Type specific (ABO matched – takes ~15 minutes)
- Fully cross matched (takes ~1 hour)
- Massive transfusion pack (packed red blood cells plus clotting factors)

Disability

Assess disability for:
- Alterations in conscious level (AVPU – Box 24.10)
- Pupillary response to light and accommodation
- Obvious lateralising signs or focal neurology

Box 24.10 AVPU scale

- **A**lert
- Responds to **V**oice
- Responds to **P**ain
- **U**nresponsive

Exposure/Environment

- External signs of injury
- Environmental factors (remove chemicals/heat, rewarm, etc.)
- Check blood sugar and core temperature, if not already done

Special populations

- Elderly (different physiology/pharmacology)
- Paediatric (different psychology/physiology, distressed parents)
- Obstetric (different physiology, slightly altered priorities)
- Athletes (different physiology)

Secondary survey

- Thjs only takes place once the primary survey is completed and the patient is stabilised
- Take an 'AMPLE' history (Box 24.11) and head to toe examination
- Timing and adjuncts will depend on the patient and facilities

---

Box 24.11 AMPLE history

A	Allergies
M	Medications
P	Past medical history/pregnancy
L	Last meal
E	Events surrounding incident

Avoiding complications

The following simple things can be done to avoid late complications:

- Avoid hypoxia
- Maintain normovolaemia
- Normalise $PaCO_2$
- Minimise risk of raised intracranial pressure
- Avoid hypothermia
- Consider early administration of clotting factors

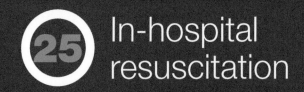

In-hospital resuscitation

25

NB Try to prevent cardiac arrest – 80% of patients who have a cardiac arrest in hospital display adverse signs prior to collapse.

- Cardiopulmonary resuscitation (CPR) is an emergency procedure performed during a cardiac arrest in an attempt to re-establish circulation and breathing
- The Resuscitation Council (UK) in-hospital algorithm (Figure 25.1) provides guidance for in-hospital resuscitation
- CPR is performed to keep a patient alive until a reversible cause can be treated and advanced emergency care can be provided
- With most patients displaying adverse signs prior to cardiac arrest, the recognition of acute illness, together with effective treatment and appropriate management following the ABCDE approach to prevent deterioration is paramount

Procedure

Safety
- Ensure it is safe to approach
- Don gloves, aprons, etc. as soon as it is practical to do so
- Check for and remove hazards, e.g. bed table, trailing electrical cables, IV fluids stand
- Remember the Resuscitation Council (UK) guidelines for safer handling in resuscitation

Medical Student Survival Skills: The Acutely Ill Patient, First Edition. Philip Jevon, Konnur Ramkumar, and Emma Jenkinson.
© 2020 John Wiley & Sons Ltd. Published 2020 by John Wiley & Sons Ltd.
Companion website: www.wiley.com/go/jevon/medicalstudent

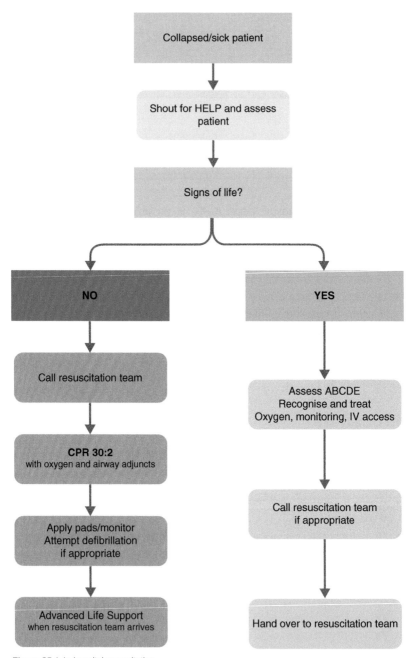

Figure 25.1 In-hospital resuscitation.

Check for response

- Gently shake the shoulders and ask loudly, 'Are you all right?' (Figure 25.2)
- If the patient responds, reassess following the ABCDE approach (see Chapter 1)
- If the patient does not respond, call out for help/pull the emergency buzzer (Figure 25.3), get the patient flat, open the airway, and check for signs of normal breathing

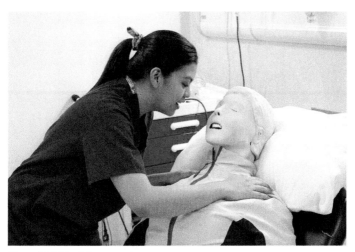

Figure 25.2 Check for responsiveness.

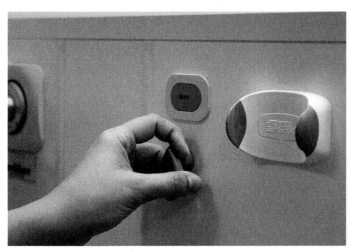

Figure 25.3 Summon help from colleagues.

Check for signs of life

- Open the airway: head tilt/chin lift (jaw thrust if cervical spine injury is suspected)
- Look, listen, and feel for signs of normal breathing for no longer than 10 seconds (Figure 25.4)

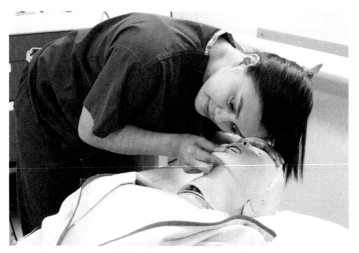

Figure 25.4 Perform head tilt/chin lift and check for signs of normal breathing.

 Common mistakes and pitfalls

Agonal breathing (occasional gasps, slow, laboured, or noisy breathing) is common in the first few minutes following a cardiac arrest. Do not mistake this for normal breathing.

- If the patient is breathing normally, perform ABCDE assessment, call for help, and escalate if necessary. Consider using the recovery position
- If the patient is not breathing normally, start chest compressions while colleagues alert the cardiac arrest team and fetch a cardiac arrest trolley and defibrillator

Alert the cardiac arrest team

- Alert the cardiac arrest team following local protocols. This usually involves calling 2222 and advising the switchboard of the emergency (cardiac arrest) and location (Figure 25.5)

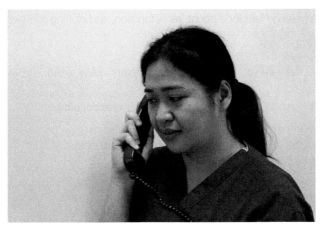

Figure 25.5 Summon cardiac arrest team: usually call 2222.

- Ensure the cardiac arrest team have access – sometimes access doors may be security locked

Chest compressions
- Ensure the bed is at a suitable height to perform chest compressions. The patient should be level with the rescuer's knee to mid-thigh region
- Place the heel of one hand on the centre of the patient's chest and the heel of the other hand on top; interlock the fingers, lifting them off the rib cage
- Ensure your arms are straight, elbows locked, and start performing chest compressions at a rate of 100–120 min^{-1} at a depth of 5–6 cm (Figure 25.6)

 NB Allow the chest to completely recoil after each compression otherwise venous return can be compromised.

- Ensure chest compression/relaxation times are approximately equal and minimise interruptions to chest compressions
- Deliver chest compressions to ventilations at a ratio of 30 : 2 (Figure 25.7). In-hospital chest compressions are typically performed continuously until a self-inflating bag device is available for ventilations

Ventilations
- As soon as the self-inflating bag arrives, attach oxygen at a flow rate of 10–15 l min^{-1} and ideally insert an airway device, e.g. oropharyngeal airway or i-gel (more experienced practitioners may insert a tracheal tube)

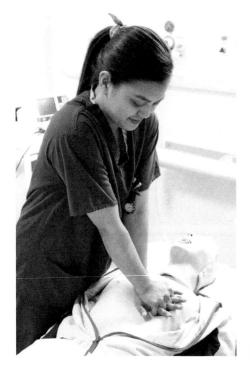

Figure 25.6 Perform chest compressions.

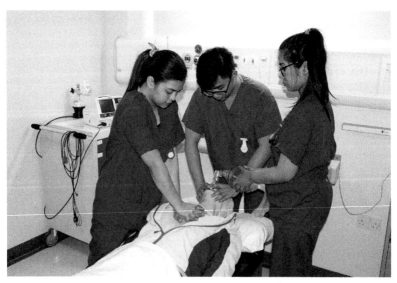

Figure 25.7 CPR: 30 chest compressions to 2 ventilations.

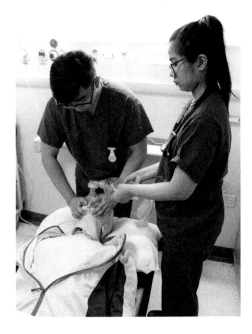

Figure 25.8 Two person technique for bag–valve–mask ventilation.

- Ensure the airway is open and there is an adequate seal between the mask and the patient's mouth (Figure 25.8)
- Stop chest compressions and deliver two ventilations, each over 1 second and then continue chest compressions and ventilations at a ratio of 30:2

Defibrillation (if required)
- Once the defibrillator arrives, switch it on, and use in automated external defibrillator (AED) mode
- Attach large adhesive defibrillation pads to the patient's bare chest – one to the right of the sternum below the clavicle and the other in the mid-axillary line approximately level with the V6 electrocardiogram (ECG) electrode, avoiding breast tissue

NB Chest compressions should continue while pads are being attached.

- Once the defibrillator starts to analyse the ECG, ensure cadiopulmonary resuscitation (CPR) is stopped. If a shock is required the defibrillator will charge up and advise you to shock (semi-automatic)

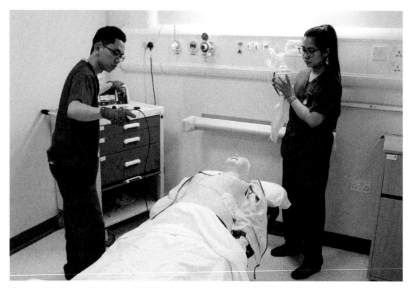

Figure 25.9 Automated external defibrillation: ensure everyone is clear of the patient.

- Before pressing the shock button, ensure everyone is clear of the patient and that the oxygen is removed 1 m (Figure 25.9)
- After delivering the shock continue with CPR for 2 minutes

Cardiac arrest rhythms – shockable

Ventricular fibrillation

- In ventricular fibrillation (VF) various groups of cells within the ventricles are depolarising and repolarising in an uncoordinated, random, and chaotic way
- This results in insufficient contraction of the left ventricle and insufficient cardiac output to produce a pulse

Ventricular tachycardia

- In ventricular tachycardia (VT) cells within the ventricles are initiating the action potential at a fast rate, usually 120–200 bpm
- In some cases this rate may be so fast that it does not allow sufficient time for adequate ventricular filling, resulting in a reduction in cardiac output. If this reduction is dramatic enough, the casualty may not have a palpable pulse; the rhythm is described as 'pulseless ventricular tachycardia'

Cardiac arrest rhythms – non-shockable

Asystole

- Asystole is often described as a 'straight line'. However, in reality the line is rarely (if ever) straight
- Occasionally P waves may be seen
- This rhythm is known by a number of different names including ventricular standstill and P wave asystole

Pulseless electrical activity

- Pulseless electrical activity (PEA) occurs in patients who have organised cardiac electrical activity in the absence of any palpable pulses
- There will always be an underlying cause to PEA

Potentially reversible causes: The four 'H's and four 'T's

Potentially reversible or aggravating causes for the cardiac arrest should be considered and where possible appropriate treatment initiated. The main reversible causes are identified as the four 'H's and four 'T's, using their initial letter.

- Hypoxia
- Hypovolaemia
- Hyperkalaemia, hypokalaemia, hypoglycaemia, hypocalcaemia, acidaemia, and other metabolic disorders
- Hypothermia
- Tension pneumothorax
- Tamponade
- Toxins
- Thrombosis (pulmonary or coronary)

Hypoxia

- Any casualty in cardiac arrest will have some degree of hypoxia
- Oxygen should be administered using as high a concentration as possible
- Check regularly to make sure that any oxygen tubing used is connected securely to the oxygen flow meter

- Oxygen cylinders found on many cardiac arrest trolleys have limited capacity. Check the cylinder pressure gauge regularly to ensure that the cylinder is not empty
- Always use a central supply of oxygen via an outlet in the wall by the casualty's bed whenever possible

Hypovolaemia

- Hypovolaemia is usually due to severe haemorrhage. Intravenous fluids should be administered rapidly and, if necessary, arrangements made for urgent surgery
- Although there has been a great deal of debate as to the most appropriate fluids to give in such circumstances, it is suggested that there is no advantage in using a colloid so either sodium chloride 0.9% or Hartmann's solution should be used

Hyperkalaemia, hypokalaemia, and other metabolic disorders

- The casualty's medical history may suggest an abnormality, with appropriate tests confirming the levels
- Treatment should be directed at returning any abnormal values to normal limits; 10 ml of 10% calcium chloride or calcium gluconate can be used in the presence of hyperkalaemia and hypocalcaemia

Hypothermia

- If hypothermia is suspected, the casualty's body temperature must be checked using a low reading thermometer. Hypothermia is defined as a core body temperature below 35 °C and is further classified as being mild (32–35 °C), moderate (30–32 °C), or severe (< 30 °C)
- Emphasis is placed on rewarming the casualty, whilst maintaining CPR throughout. Various options are available for use for a patient in cardiac arrest including warming intravenous fluids, and placing warm fluid into the casualty's bladder, peritoneal (abdominal) cavity, or pleural (thoracic) cavity
- Many drugs and other treatment options such as defibrillation may be ineffective at temperatures below 30 °C and careful consideration needs to be given to the use of these at such low temperatures

Tension pneumothorax

- A tension pneumothorax may be the result of trauma to the chest, a severe asthma attack, positive pressure ventilation, including the use of a bag-valve-mask, or following some medical procedures such as the insertion of a central venous line

- Initial management of a tension pneumothorax involves the insertion of a large bore cannula into the 2nd intercostal space in the mid-clavicular line (needle thoracocentesis). The casualty will also require the insertion of a chest drain

Tamponade

- A cardiac tamponade results from fluid or blood entering the pericardial space. As more fluid enters the space, more pressure is exerted on the heart until it is physically unable to beat, resulting in little or no cardiac output
- A cardiac tamponade is difficult to diagnose, especially during a cardiac arrest. A cardiac tamponade should be considered in any casualty in cardiac arrest following penetrating chest trauma, and chest or cardiac surgery. A needle pericardiocentesis should be considered

Toxins

- Consideration should be given to the possibility that the casualty has a specific history of accidental or deliberate poisoning. Specific antidotes may be available
- Many hospital emergency departments have databases outlining the appropriate treatment options for many drugs, plants, or other chemicals and toxic substances that may be ingested. Similarly, the National Poisons Information Service (www.npis.org) offers such advice
- CPR must be continued in the pulseless casualty whilst any other treatment is undertaken

Thrombosis

- The most likely cause is a large pulmonary embolism
- Thrombolytic drugs should be considered. However, thrombolytic drugs may take up to 90 minutes to be effective and must only be used if it is appropriate to continue resuscitative attempts for this duration

References

Bernal, W., Auzinger, G., Dhawan, A., and Wendon, J. (2010). Acute liver failure. *Lancet* 376: 190–201.

Blatchford, O., Murray, W.R., and Blatchford, M. (2000). A risk score to predict need for treatment for upper gastrointestinal haemorrhage. *Lancet* 356 (9238): 1318–1321.

Rockall, T.A., Logan, R.F., Devlin, H.B., and Northfield, T.C. (1996). Risk assessment after acute upper gastrointestinal haemorrhage. *Gut* 38 (3): 316–321.

Rutherford, R.B. (2009). Clinical staging of acute limb ischaemia as the basis for choice of revascularization method: when and how to intervene. *Seminars in Vascular Surgery* 22 (1): 5–9.

Slack, A. and Wendon, J. (2011). Acute liver failure. *Clinical Medicine* 11 (3): 254–258.

Index

Note: Page numbers in *italics* refer to figures.
Page numbers in **bold** refer to tables.

Medical Student Survival Skills: The Acutely Ill Patient, First Edition. Philip Jevon,
Konnur Ramkumar, and Emma Jenkinson.
© 2020 John Wiley & Sons Ltd. Published 2020 by John Wiley & Sons Ltd.
Companion website: www.wiley.com/go/jevon/medicalstudent